INNER CLEANSING

*How to Free Yourself from
Joint-Muscle-Artery-Circulation Sludge*

OTHER BOOKS BY THE AUTHOR

Health Tonics, Elixirs and Potions for the Look and Feel of Youth
Natural Hormones: The Secret of Youthful Health
Health Secrets from the Orient
Magic Enzymes: Key to Youth and Health
The Miracle of Organic Vitamins for Better Health
Miracle Protein: Secret of Natural Cell-Tissue Rejuvenation
All-Natural Pain Relievers
The New Enzyme-Catalyst Diet: Amazing Way to Quick, Permanent Weight Loss
Brand Name Handbook of Protein, Calories and Carbohydrates
Slimfasting—the Quick "Pounds Off" Way to Youthful Slimness
Healing and Revitalizing Your Vital Organs
Miracle Rejuvenation Energizers
Encyclopedia of Power Foods for Health and Longer Life
Helping Yourself with New Enzyme Catalyst Health Secrets
Catalytic Hormones, Key to Extraordinary Weight Loss

INNER CLEANSING

How to Free Yourself from
Joint-Muscle-Artery-Circulation Sludge

CARLSON WADE

Parker Publishing Company   West Nyack, New York

Library of Congress Cataloging in Publication Data

Wade, Carlson.
  Inner cleansing.

  Includes index.
  1. Self-care, Health.   2. Diet therapy.
I. Title.
RA776.95.W33   1983   615.8'8   82-18972

ISBN 0-13-465583-4
ISBN 0-13-465575-3 {PBK}

Printed in the United States of America

DEDICATION

To Your Sparkling Clean and Youthful New Body

FOREWORD BY A DOCTOR OF MEDICINE

Suddenly, here is a bright new world of youthful health. It is yours, ready for the taking.

This was my immediate reaction when I read Carlson Wade's latest book, *Inner Cleansing: How to Free Yourself from Joint-Muscle-Artery-Circulation Sludge*. It is a dynamic key to self-rejuvenation from head to toe.

This leading medical reporter has discovered the basic causes of hundreds of ailments, which include: premature aging to allergies, digestive disorders to cardiovascular problems, overweight to sluggish circulation. All are thoroughly described, and contain amazingly simple but speedily effective home remedies. This is a lifesaving book!

Carlson Wade calls the problem "internal sludge." He is correct. It is this invisible internal accumulation of toxic wastes that can cause erosion of your body and mind. It is the major cause of aging. So I am glad that Carlson Wade has "unmasked" this sneak thief of health. I highly recommend the programs that help you wash pollution right out of your system so you can become sparklingly clean and youthfully healthy . . . at any age.

The great joy here is that so many of these easy-to-follow home programs give rejuvenation results within minutes! I have seen this myself. Carlson Wade presents simple programs that can solve a lifetime of problems immediately. And all are natural. *No* drugs. *No* medicines. *No* hospitalization. You'll never have a sick day. This is truly a miracle in rejuvenation and healing. And it works!

Inner Cleansing is the most helpful book on total healing that I have yet to see. Use it. Discover how it can make you look and feel young again . . . forever.

H. W. Holderby, M.D.

7

WHAT THIS BOOK WILL DO FOR YOU

This book was written to alert you to an "invisible" threat to your youthful health. We identify it as "body pollution."

This internal pollution is so deceptive, its gnawing presence is hardly noticed until you start to develop one "hopeless" condition after another. Examples of these conditions range from arthritis to sagging skin, from high blood pressure to clogged arteries, from chronic indigestion to undesirable overweight. This means the aging process has taken root inside your body. Something must be done, and quickly.

This book will tell you about the latest bio-nutritional discoveries of "body pollution." It will show how you can reverse the tide and rid yourself completely of this threat to your youthfulness.

All together, in one comprehensive volume, at your finger tips for immediate use and help, are easy-to-follow programs. They can save your life. They can help add years of vitality to your life. They can restore youth to your body and mind!

This book shows how you can cleanse yourself of almost any ailment—right at home. There are *no* drugs, *no* expensive hospitalization costs, and *no* cumbersome equipment. Many of the sludge-cleansing programs are totally free. Some require everyday ingredients that are probably in your pantry right now. All of these programs work swiftly. They search out, dissolve, and then wash away internal sediment that might otherwise deteriorate your vital systems.

Stiffened by arthritis? Troubled with cholesterol-clogged arteries? Wrinkled skin? Nagging stomach disorders? Stubborn overweight? Draining allergies? Cardiovascular distress? Blood sludge? Feel aged because of "muscular stiffness"?

Then get ready for sets of easy-to-follow programs (they're fun, too!) that will free your body from pollutants and make you feel young and clean on both the inside and outside. This book will help you whether these conditions just started or have plagued you for a long time.

Concerned about the side effects of drugs? About the uncertainties of surgery? The spiralling costs of constant medical care? Then this book holds special value. The programs described are *all natural,* and can be done right at home. Often, they cost just pennies (yes, pennies!). Most importantly, they give you *fast* and permanent healing in a short time. In many cases, you'll see and feel the rejuvenation within minutes! And that is just the start of these benefits.

When these discoveries begin to heal you, say goodbye to hundreds of formerly "hopeless" problems. Discover the joys of looking and feeling young and healthy forever. Reason? This book unmasks the "unknown" basic cause of aging and illness: *internal pollution.* It shows you how to uproot, loosen, and wash away this sludge and discover the joys of vigorous, youthful health.

How soon will you enjoy this "fountain of youth"? Almost immediately, when you turn the page . . .

Carlson Wade

Contents

Foreword by a Doctor of Medicine 7

What This Book Will Do for You 9

1 Free Yourself from "Arthritis Pain" with Biological
Washing 19

Toxic Waste Overload—Arthritis Cause—19 • "Wash Away
Arthritis" with This Two-Day Raw Food Plan—20 • Overcome
"Hopeless" Arthritis on a Nightshade-Free Program—21 • The
Oil That Cleans Away Arthritis Sludge—22 • The Tiny Ancient
Vegetable That Conquers Arthritis Pain—23 • How to "Steam
Clean" Your Body and End Arthritis Pain—25 • Nine Ways to
Cleanse Your Body with Stretching—26 • Biological Washing:
Key to Arthritis Freedom—28

2 The Cholesterol Cleansing Way to Longer Life 29

Cholesterol—Toxic Sludge—29 • Everyday Foods That Scrub
Away Stubborn Cholesterol Wastes—30 • Lecithin Washes
Away Cholesterol Sludge—31 • Pectin for Balance of HDL-LDL
Reactions—32 • Three Easy Ways to Boost Cell-Washing
Actions—35 • Ten Ways to Protect Against Cholesterol
Overload—36 • Your Cholesterol-Watching Chart—37

3 "Forever Young" Skin Through Catalytic Cleansing ... 41

Problem: Skin-Aging Cellulite—41 • Free Your Body of Cellulite
in Six Steps—43 • Catalytic Skin Cleansers for Common and
Uncommon Disorders—46 • Catalytic Cleansing—Baby Skin at
Any Age—49

4 How to Balance Your Blood Pressure with Internal Washing **51**

What Does "Blood Pressure" Mean?—51 • Beware Prolonged Hypertension—52 • Toxic Waste Overload—Root Cause of Runaway Blood Pressure—52 • Garlic Washes Your Arteries, Balances Your Blood Pressure—53 • Garlic + Onions = Healthy Blood Pressure—54 • The Low-Salt Way to Waste-Free Arteries and Normal Pressure—55 • Six Ways to Maintain Clean Arteries and Balanced Blood Pressure—56 • The "Snack" That Controls Blood Pressure—57 • Wash Away Hypertension . . . Without Delay—58

5 How to Revitalize Your Digestive System for Total Youth   61

How to Wash Away the "Glue" That Creates Constipation—61 • Potassium: The Mineral That Opens Up Tight Intestinal Organs—62 • The 25¢ Fruit That Causes Swift Waste-Washing—62 • The "Miracle Salad" That Rejuvenates Digestive System—63 • How to Wash Away the Irritants of Indigestion—64 • How to Wash Away the Pain of Ulcers—66

6 Foods That Wash Away Overweight **69**

Cellular Overload—Real Cause of Overweight—69 • Food Enzymes Wash Away Fatty Wastes—70 • 23 Foods That Wash Away Your Overweight—71 • Two Simple Steps That Protect Against Cellular Overweight—74 • Say "No" to These Waste-Causing Foods—75

7 Say Goodbye to Allergies with Cellular Washing **77**

Allergy-Causing Internal Pollution—77 • One-Day Juice Fast = Freedom from Allergies—78 • Clean Up Your Lifestyle and Clean Up Your Breathing Organs—79 • Alternate Nostril-Breathing Technique for Internal Cleansing—82 • Whistle Your Way to Cleaner Lungs—83

8 How to Supercharge Your Heart with Youthful Power . . . While You Sleep! 85

How Toxemia Can Contribute to Heart Distress—85 • Internal Washing Protects Against Heart Attack—86 • "Waste-Forming" Vs. "Waste-Cleaning" Foods—86 • Cleanse Your Heart While You Sleep—87 • Garlic: Amazing Total Heart Cleanser—88 • The Super-Cleansing Food That Doubles Your Heart Power—89 • Stimulate Internal Cleansing in Minutes—90 • An Onion a Day Keeps Your Heart Doctor Away—91 • "All-Natural Heart Cleansing Tonic"—92

9 Miracle Power Foods for Dynamic Circulation 95

How Foods Boost Youthful Circulation—95 • One-Day Grape Juice Fast = Forever Young Circulation—96 • "Early Morning Circulation Booster"—97 • Limit (or Eliminate) These Circulation-Blocking Foods—98 • The Clot-Cleansing Vitamin That May Save Your Life—99 • "Triple Circulation Pick-Up Elixir"—101

10 How to "Unlock" and "Release" Wastes for Freedom from "Aging Stiffness" 103

Wash Out Lactic Acid for Greater Joint-Muscle Flexibility—104 • The Food That Washes Wastes and Rejuvenates Joints—104 • How to Use Lecithin for Speedy Joint-Muscle Energy—105 • "Instant Power Potion"—105 • How to Ventilate Your Joints for Greater Mobility—106 • Garlic: Dynamic Waste-Washer—108 • How to Steam Wastes Out of Your Joints—108

11 Cleanse Your Organs for Total Revitalization 111

Less Sugar + Less Strain = Stronger Eyesight—111 • Less Cooking = Less Internal Wastes—113 • How Vitamin C + Bioflavonoids Wash Away Cataract Debris—114 • Better Hearing with Cleaner Ears—116 • How to Cleanse and Energize Your Ears for Super-Hearing—117 • The Low-Fat Way to Improved Hearing—118 • Keep Your Kidneys Clean for Internal

Rejuvenation—118 • The Berry Juice That Dissolves Kidney Gravel—120 • Washing Your Liver for Total Health—120 • How to Keep Your Gall Bladder in Tiptop Condition—121 • The Food That Helps Wash Away Gall Bladder Wastes—122 • Plain Water Helps Wash Away Bladder Crystals—122

12 How to Cleanse Your Bloodstream and Enrich Your Entire Body **125**

The Everyday Food That Creates a Sparkling Clean Bloodstream—126 • How to Wash and "Iron" Your Blood Cells for Super Health—127 • Balloon Breathing Builds Stronger Blood Cells—129 • "Triple-Action Blood-Washing Potion"—130

13 Cleanse Your Arteries and Enjoy a "Second Youth" **133**

Waste Overload = Clogged Arteries—133 • Arteriosclerosis—Excess Sludge Accumulation—134 • Can Food Make You Feel Young Forever?—135 • Results Are Cleansing—136 • How Simple Exercises Cause Artery Scrubbing in Days—137 • Why Triglyceride Control Is Important to Arterial Youthfulness—138 • The Cleansing Power of Garlic—139 • The Quick Way to Correct "Metabolic Sluggishness" and "Smoggy Oxygen"—139

14 How Body Motions Wash Away Stubborn Aches and Pains **143**

Regular Body Motions Protect Against Recurring Aches—143 • Easy Body Motions Cleanse Away Bursitis Toxemia—144 • Easy Leg-Ercises to Melt Away Toxemia-Caused Cramps—146 • Casting Out "Phantom Aches"—147 • Washing (the Insides) of Your Feet for Freedom from Aches—149

15 How to De-Age Your Cells and Make Your Body Brand New Again **151**

Clean Cells = Total Rejuvenation—151 • The Vitamin That Restores "Young Power" to Your Cells—152 • Vitamin C

Rebuilds "Aging" Skin Cells—153 • Why Animal Fats Are Harmful to Your Cells—155 • How Fish Oils De-Age Your Cells and Add Years to Your Life—156 • How Fish Oils Improve Lymph Flow—157 • Rebuild Lymphatic System, Regenerate Cells, Rejuvenate Body—159

16 **The 10¢ Magic Food That Performs Total Cleansing Within Hours** 161

Meet This Dynamic Cleanser—161 • Fiber: How It Digests, Cleanses, Heals—162 • Decreased Transit Time Is Secret of Fiber's Magic—162 • Everyday Food Sources of Cleansing Fiber—164 • The Single Most Concentrated Source of Cleansing Fiber—164 • Fiber in Selected Foods—165 • "Morning Bran Booster Tonic"—167 • Discover Wheat Germ: Cell Cleanser Supreme—167 • How to Use Bran and Wheat Germ for Daily Cell Cleansing—168

17 **The Raw Juice Way to Super Cleansing and Healthy Youth . . . At Any Age** 171

Cause of Aging: Cellular Grime—171 • Raw Juices Are Swift in Cellular Regeneration—172 • Juices Work Faster Than Whole Foods—172 • Seven Cleansing-Rejuvenating Powers of Fresh Juices—173 • Simple Juice-Taking Program—175 • Tasty Juices for Healing of Common Ailments—175

18 **A Treasury of Cleansing Programs for Common and Uncommon Everyday Problems** 179

How Juices Give You Quick Cleansing and Better Health—183 • Summary—186

Index 187

INNER CLEANSING

*How to Free Yourself from
Joint-Muscle-Artery-Circulation Sludge*

CHAPTER *1*

Free Yourself from "Arthritis Pain" with Biological Washing

To free yourself from arthritis, you must correct the cause of this painful, oft-crippling ailment. By using simple programs that initiate "biological washing," you uproot, dislodge, and eliminate internal congestion. This "washing" frees your system and skeletal structure from toxic wastes—those irritating, grating, inflammation-causing leftover accumulations that are largely responsible for arthritic distress. Once these cell-clogging wastes have been washed out of your system, your skeletal-muscular network functions smoothly, without blockage that otherwise is responsible for the stiffness and pain that grows worse as toxic wastes continue accumulating.

TOXIC WASTE OVERLOAD—ARTHRITIS CAUSE

What Are Toxic Wastes? These are leftover fragments from incompleted digestive processes; they are also remnants from improper foods, refined products, and harsh chemical additives. Toxic wastes become stored throughout your body, in all glands, in all cellular spaces, and circulate throughout your bloodstream. They cling together, creating barriers that prevent free movement of your limbs and free muscular ability. This is the forerunner of arthritic-like distress. Internally, you are "clogged" or "choked" with these toxic wastes. If not washed out, they continue growing in size until they cause changes in your joint structure, inflammation takes hold, and you fall victim to what is considered to be advancing arthritis. Must this happen? Not if you are able to begin simple, swift *internal washing* with everyday foods and at-home programs that can wash away this pain-causing sludge.

"WASH AWAY ARTHRITIS" WITH THIS TWO-DAY RAW FOOD PLAN

Fresh raw fruits and vegetables (and their fresh juices) are highly concentrated sources of catalytic enzymes. These are protein-like substances that start cell-scrubbing action to break down, dissolve, and ultimately eliminate the toxic waste materials that irritate your joint-muscle system and erupt into arthritis distress. Almost "overnight" fresh fruits and vegetables begin the biological washing of your debris-laden organs and systems. Once free of these blockages, your joints and muscles can move without obstruction. Increased flexibility and freedom from arthritis is your reward for internal cleansing.

Simple Two-Day Raw Food Plan   Set aside two days per week for this internal cleansing program. During these days, consume nothing but raw foods. *Example:* Eat fresh fruits in any desired combination such as fresh fruit juices for breakfast, a raw vegetable platter with a vegetable juice for lunch. Dinner could be another raw vegetable meal and any desired vegetable juice.

Benefit: Catalytic enzymes are now able to devote full activity to dissolving the sludge that has accumulated throughout your body. Working swiftly, the enzymes break down these plaque-like molecules and prepare them for elimination. The wrongdoings of the rest of the week can be counteracted with this simple two-day plan. *Suggestion:* To protect your joints and muscles from toxic waste overload, eliminate your intake of refined and processed foods. This helps to maintain a more youthful metabolism and a system that is healthfully free of arthritis-causing cellular waste material.

"Body Spring Cleaning" Ends Lifetime Arthritis Pain

Pain-wracked fingers that could hardly hold a spoon, stiff back that made getting up from a chair or bed a painful ordeal, and knees that refused to bend at will, so depressed Edna J., that she felt there was no alternative but a hospital or sanitarium. A nutrition-minded nurse read her tests and charts and recognized the symptoms of sludge-laden joints and muscles. She suggested that Edna J. follow a "body spring cleaning" program for just two or even three days weekly that called for eating only raw foods and raw juices in any quantity or combination throughout the day. She was to eat nothing processed and nothing cooked. Edna J. was so desperate, she would try anything. By the end of the second day, she felt her fingers becoming more flexible. She could even bend her knees. Encouraged, she continued on the program for five consecutive days. At the end of the five days she could bend at the waist, do usual housework, even go bowling . . . and win! This simple program ended her lifetime arthritis pain. To maintain "body spring cleaning" all year long, Edna J. goes on a tasty raw food plan for two days every week. She now has the flexibility of a youngster. She feels "saved" from the discouragement of confinement in a sanitarium . . . thanks to this cellular cleansing program.

OVERCOME "HOPELESS" ARTHRITIS ON A NIGHTSHADE-FREE PROGRAM

A group of foods comprises the nightshade family. These are crop plants that ordinarily offer good nutrition, but for certain people, they become antagonistic. These nightshade foods contain substances which block enzymes in your muscles from cleansing and metabolizing waste materials.

Problem: The nightshade foods release toxins which initiate the stimulation of *solanine*. This is a crystalline alkaloid which festers in the joints and muscles and eventually causes enervation (lowered resistance) and the onset of arthritic distress. Certain people are especially sensitive to even small amounts of this solanine. Furthermore, if your metabolism is sluggish, the solanine accumulates and creates a sludge-like barrier in your joint-muscle cells. Blockage is felt in the form of stiff joints. Pain, unhappily, is the symptom most often experienced. This can all be traced back to the sensitivity to solanine.

Solution: If you experience stubborn stiffness that does not respond to the usual internal washing programs, then you may be allergic to the nightshade group of foods. *Simple Plan:* Eliminate tomatoes, potatoes, green or red peppers, and eggplants in any form from your food program. These are four foods that are high in substances that boost pain-causing solanine in your system. Doing this may well bring about an end to your arthritic distress.

No-Nightshade Diet = No Arthritis Pain In Eight Days

A victim of osteoarthritis (degenerative joint disease) for ten years, farmer Morton A. faced serious financial losses by being unable to work his land. The expense of hired hands made it a losing proposition. Medications gave him side effects worse than the stiffness and debilitation caused by his osteoarthritis. He needed help badly. He received it from a food technologist at the nutrition laboratory connected with the local university hospital. Morton A. was tested, found to be allergic (yes, allergic!) to the nightshade group of foods. The allergic symptoms erupted into osteoarthritis. Morton A.'s joints and muscles had toxic waste overload; cells were encrusted with debris from faulty metabolism of the *solanine*, stimulated by the substances in the nightshade foods. Hence, the arthritis pain.

Morton A. made one simple change: he avoided the four nightshade foods listed above in any form. His reward was, within three days he had increased flexibility of his arms and legs. At the end of the sixth day, he could do routine chores with the vitality of a youngster. By the eighth day, he was so energetic and alive he released his hired hands and did all the work himself as before. Not only was his farm saved from financial disaster—he was saved from crippling confinement. Just avoiding these four foods made him free from arthritis and feeling young again!

THE OIL THAT CLEANS AWAY "ARTHRITIS SLUDGE"

You must remember cod liver oil if your parents gave it to you as a youngster throughout the winter to help protect you against colds. Haven't taken it in years? Then rediscover it. Cod liver oil is a prime source of essential fatty acids which are able to cleanse away the sludge from your joints and muscles. These EFA substances, as they are called, also help wash away sediment from your bloodstream. This starts the needed internal washing that helps you enjoy clean and flexible joints and muscles.

Cleansing Power of Cod Liver Oil   The highly volatile EFA substances have the ability to penetrate the inner recesses of your joints and muscles so that this vital cleansing can occur.

Unique Cleansing Power: Cod liver oil contains a unique essential fatty acid known as *eicosapentaenoic acid*. This jawbreaker of a substance (called EPA) is propelled into your blood vessels. Here, EPA becomes an *anti-aggregating* substance, able to break down blood sludge and prepare it for elimination. This is a unique cleansing power, and it is possible with cod liver oil.

How to Take: Mix two tablespoons of cod liver oil with two tablespoons of either citrus fruit juice or cool milk. Take this four-tablespoon combination in the morning, two hours *before* breakfast. For severe arthritis distress, take this same four-tablespoon combo some five hours *after* your final meal of the day. *Tip:* Be sure to shake the ingredients thoroughly in a screw-top jar before drinking. Assimilated, they work more effectively in cleansing arthritis sludge.

Benefit: The ascorbic acid in the citrus juice activates the EPA factor in the cod liver oil and causes an invigoration of its anti-aggregating reaction. (If taken in milk, the minerals and protein give more strength. You may want to take it in juice in the morning and milk at night for a double-barrelled, sludge-washing reaction.) If taken this way daily, you will help maintain clean blood and joints and muscles and protect yourself against arthritis.

"Oiled Joints" Become Youthful Within a Week

Martha K. grimaced with pain whenever she had to reach to a high shelf in her kitchen cupboard. At times, simple vacuuming so twisted her back, she was bedridden for the rest of the day. She humorously called her joints "dry." She might have surrendered to inevitable crippling had not an orthomolecular physician (who was nutrition-minded) diagnosed her problem as blood sludge. He put her on the cod liver oil regimen. Almost immediately, her joints had less inflammation and reduced swelling. She could move with greater agility. By the end of just one week, she could do her daily household chores without any pain. Her "oiled joints" had made her young again, thanks to the EPA action that lowered the sedimentation rate of her blood. In effect, the EPA action cleansed her joints—"oiled" them— so that she could say goodbye to arthritis.

THE TINY ANCIENT VEGETABLE THAT CONQUERS ARTHRITIS PAIN

For thousands of years, one vegetable has been hailed as a wonder food with miracle healing benefits. Today, this tiny vegetable has the amazing power of bringing about internal cleansing as well as freedom from arthritis. What is it?

Garlic!

A member of the onion family, garlic is unique because it contains antibacterial and antifungal properties that make it a total body cleanser. In modern times, garlic has emerged as a power food with important arthritis-fighting properties.

Secret Pain-Ending Power of Garlic   The power of garlic as a pain-killer may be considered "secret" because for many years this knowledge was confined largely within the medical profession, and not known about in lay circles. So it is with great excitement that the benefits of garlic are now being made available to all. Here they are:

Garlic gives off an unusual type of ultraviolet reaction called mitogenetic radiation. These emissions are called "Gurwitch rays" after the European electrobiologist who first reported their pain-killing powers. These same Gurwitch rays are able to dislodge toxic wastes from their encrusted blockages and then prepare them for elimination. This helps stimulate new cell growth and provide a rejuvenative response to all body functions.

Brings Down Inflammation, Soothes Pain   When you consume garlic, your digestive system, through enzyme activity, will extract a substance from the garlic called *allisotin*. Your enzymes then use allisotin, which employs a scrubbing action to cool down the in-flammation that is the bane of rheumatoid and other types of arthritis. The same allisotin, from eaten garlic, is also used to soothe pain by washing away the grating sand-like wastes that cling to your vital joints, muscles and related organs. In so doing, garlic, via the allisotin action, is able to help you conquer arthritis pain.

How to Take Garlic: Potency is highest in the garlic bulb itself. Take three cloves, chop them finely, and add to a raw vegetable salad or any sandwich. Add diced garlic to a bowl of soup. Use garlic for any stew, casserole, or baked dish. Chew a garlic clove or two daily. Mask the odor with parsley, of course, and you'll feel the cleansing action almost at once.

arlic Odor? There's no need to be a social outcast.
: this basic fact: the odor is noticed only when you
:. There is no odor in *cooked* garlic. If you take raw
ze the odor by chewing parsley at the same time. Or,
ving licorice (chemical-free from health store), or
innamon stick, or some cloves. (All are available at
You'll sweeten your breath and be socially accept-
able as a garlic eater. You'll also become more flexible in your joints
and muscles, thanks to garlic's ability to cleanse your body.

HOW TO "STEAM CLEAN" YOUR BODY AND END ARTHRITIS PAIN

Hydrotherapy has long been known as an effective, all-natural way to "steam clean" the body, wash out accumulated toxins, and bring about an end to stubborn joint-muscle pain. Today, it is known as an effective way to correct toxic overload and actually end arthritis pain.

How to "Steam Clean" at Home Fill your bath with water in the temperature range of 96°F. to 103°F. Slowly immerse yourself and remain relaxed for 15 to 20 minutes. Then let the water run out of the tub. Now stand up and turn on the shower to a comfortably hot stream, gradually making it lukewarm. Stand for just five more minutes. Then turn off shower, towel dry yourself, and relax in bed. *Suggestion:* Try this "steam cleaning" body program twice daily—in the morning, then at night before going to sleep.

Toxic-Washing Benefits A leisurely soak at this temperature helps open up your billions of skin pores. While you soak, toxic wastes are steamed out of your body. At the same time, you will have soothed your nerves and relaxed their irritated state by washing away the grating wastes. When you shower, you wash away the removed toxic wastes. It is an internal (and external) method of cleansing that will be noticed when cleansed joints and muscles move with better agility.

All-Natural Internal Washing Your body temperature is controlled by a segment of your brain which serves as a thermostat.

This internal thermostat remains constant at about 98.6°F. When you soak in a hot tub, you turn up this internal thermostat. The instant reaction is for perspiration to occur. As you perspire, you create an all-natural washing! You are actually cleansing your internal organs. Accumulated wastes and debris float out with the perspiration. Just 20 minutes in the tub gives you this joint-muscle-cell scrubbing reaction. You will feel sparkling clean, and the irritants that previously caused internal erosion and subsequent pain will be gone. It's an ancient remedy that is now being hailed as an all-natural way to melt away arthritis pain.

Ends "Morning Stiffness" with Home "Steam Clean" Plan

"Morning stiffness" was more like "morning agony" for Nancy R., who found it excruciatingly painful to get out of bed when the alarm went off. As an office supervisor, she could not jeopardize her job with lateness. Yet, her stiff muscles and back made her walk like a puppet, drive like an invalid. It took her hours to get over the arthritic pains that made it difficult for her to work a computer or even apply her makeup! The company physiotherapist suggested she rid her system of pain-causing toxins with the "steam clean" bath in the morning and at night. Nancy R. felt merciful relief almost immediately. Just four days of this pleasurable and totally free pain reliever restored flexibility to her entire body. By the fifth day, she bounced out of bed with youthful agility. She was so invigorated, she was able to work overtime when she needed. And she never felt tired! The threatening arthritis pain was gone, thanks to her "steam cleaned" joints and muscles.

NINE WAYS TO CLEANSE YOUR BODY WITH STRETCHING[1]

1. *Standing Reach.* Stand erect with your feet shoulder-width apart and your arms extended over your head. Stretch as high as possible, keeping your heels on the ground. Count slowly to 15.

2. *Flexed Leg Back Stretch.* Stand erect with your feet shoulder-width apart and your arms at your sides. Slowly bend over, touching the ground between your feet. Keep your knees relaxed and flexed. Count slowly to 15 or 30. If at first you can't reach the floor, touch the top of your shoe line. Repeat 2 or 3 times.

---

[1]*Natural Health Bulletin*, Delta Group, 1101D State Road, Princeton, N.J. 08540, October 1981. Available by subscription.

3. *Alternate Knee Pull.* Lie on your back with your feet extended and hands at your sides. Pull one leg to your chest, grasp with both arms, and count slowly to 5. Repeat 7 to 10 times with each leg.

4. *Double Knee Pull.* Lie on your back with your feet extended and hands at your sides. Pull both of your legs to your chest. Lock your arms around your legs and pull your buttocks slightly off the ground. Hold and count slowly to 20 or 40. Repeat 7 to 10 times.

5. *Supine Hip Rotators.* Lie flat on your back with your legs together and your arms away from your sides, palms down. Pull your knees toward your chest and rotate your hips and legs to the left until they are touching the floor. Keep your shoulders and back flat. Repeat, rotating your hips and legs to your right side. Repeat 2 to 4 times on each side.

6. *Seated Pike Stretch.* Sit on the floor with your legs extended and your knees together. Exhale and stretch forward slowly, sliding your hands down to your ankles. Try to touch your kneecaps with your chin, keeping your legs as straight as possible. Hold position and count slowly to 5 or 10. Return to your starting position, inhaling deeply. Repeat 4 to 6 times.

7. *The Swan.* Lie on your back, with your arms at your sides, palms down. Bring your knees to your chest while elevating your hips. Bring your legs over your head, trying to touch the floor behind you. As you progress, try to touch your knees to the floor. Hold and count slowly to 5 or 10. Return to starting position, bending your knees as you lower your legs. Inhale deeply and repeat 3 to 5 times.

8. *The Dove.* Stand with your feet apart, legs slightly bent, and your hands clasped behind your back. Slowly bend at the waist while elevating your arms behind your back to the "stretching point." Count slowly to 5 or 8. Relax. Repeat.

9. *Achilles Stretch.* Stand facing a wall 2 to 3 feet away. Lean into the wall with your arms extended. Move your left leg forward one-half step, right leg backward one-half step or more. Lower your right heel to the floor. Lower your body toward the wall, stretching the heel tendon in your right leg. Count slowly to 5 or 10. Reverse leg position. Repeat, performing exercise 3 to 6 times on each leg.

Remember: There should be *no* pain when stretching. If you feel any, ease up. Progress slowly through each stretching exercise. Take deep breaths. Relax, if need be, before continuing.

BIOLOGICAL WASHING: KEY TO ARTHRITIS FREEDOM

Refresh your trillions of cells and your joints and muscles through these simple at-home and often totally free programs. They help to start the vital biological washing that scrubs away pain-causing sediment from your body's organs and helps you enjoy freedom from arthritis.

HIGHLIGHTS

1. Toxic waste overload—a cause of arthritis—needs to be biologically washed out of your system to end this painful problem.
2. Edna J. was able to "wash away arthritis" on an easy (and tasty) two-day raw food plan.
3. "Hopeless" arthritis can become healed on a nightshade-free program. The simple plan: omit four foods and solve this pain-causing problem.
4. Morton A. ended 10 years of osteoarthritis in just eight days on a no-nightshade diet.
5. Cod liver oil, if taken properly, is able to clean away "arthritis sludge."
6. Martha K. conquered crippling pain by following the cod liver oil program for just one week.
7. Garlic is a powerhouse of pain-ending ingredients.
8. "Steam clean" your body and end arthritis pain.
9. Nancy R. ended morning stiffness and afternoon pain on a totally free "steam clean" plan!
10. Stretch away arthritic stiffness and boost refreshing circulation with simple exercises that can be performed at home.

CHAPTER 2

The Cholesterol Cleansing Way
to Longer Life

With the use of everyday foods, you can help clean out cholesterol overload and maintain a level of health that will protect you against *arteriosclerosis* (hardening of the arteries) and related heart disorders. These same foods are able to loosen, dissolve and wash out accumulated cholesterol through an unusual "scrubbing" action. At the same time, by making simple substitutions, you will be able to give yourself an around-the-clock, cholesterol-cleansing metabolism, the key to a longer and healthier life.

CHOLESTEROL—TOXIC SLUDGE

What Is Cholesterol?   A tasteless, odorless, white fatty alcohol found in all animal fats and animal oils; in egg yolks; in dairy products; and in animal foods. In pure form, it is a white wax-like material that is known as toxic sludge.

Your Body Makes Cholesterol   Much of this sludge that clings to your cell walls is made by your body. The most vigorous cholesterol sludge-making factory is your very own liver, with a little help from other organs. Cholesterol is synthesized in your liver from substances derived from ingested animal-source foods. Your liver takes substances from these foods and puts them through a biological condensation process within your system, to create a compound known as *squalene*, which is the precursor of cholesterol in your body.

29

Do You Have Too Much?   You *do* need some cholesterol. It is needed for synthesis of bile acids, and is essential for digestion and absorption of fats in your intestine. Your endocrine glands use cholesterol in making valuable steroid hormones. Cholesterol is also present in your central nervous system. When faced with stress or tension, your body sends forth more cholesterol to meet the challenges of increased nerve response. So, you must have adequate cholesterol.

What's the Problem?   When your body receives or manufactures more cholesterol than it requires for everyday living, this creates an overload that may increase your risk of developing *arteriosclerosis* (thickening and narrowing of the arteries because of a decrease of elasticity of the artery walls.) It may also bring on *atherosclerosis* (a filling up and clogging of the arteries with sludge wastes such as fat and cholesterol. Your blood cannot reach most parts of your body efficiently, including your heart).

If the toxic waste cholesterol is allowed to remain and build up, thus creating internal blockages throughout your body, you run the risk of a stroke, not to mention heart trouble, as well as some forms of high blood pressure. Your body weakens and health is on the decline. All this can be traced to this toxic waste overload.

How Much Do You Need?   A doctor's blood test will tell you how much blood cholesterol you have. A rule of thumb is a reading of about 150 to 180 milligrams in 100 cc. of blood. Anything higher indicates that a cleansing program is vital.

EVERYDAY FOODS THAT SCRUB AWAY STUBBORN CHOLESTEROL WASTES

High blood cholesterol can be reversed. The accumulated plaques can be broken down, melted, and eventually washed out of your body. A set of everyday foods can scrub away the accumulated cholesterol wastes. Let's see how you can use them and enjoy a longer lifespan.

Garlic Can Unplug Your Arteries   An all-natural waste-scrubber is garlic. It is able to break down plaques that have formed inside and outside your arteries. It helps protect you against the development of atherosclerosis and heart trouble.

Scrubbing Power of Garlic   This miracle waste-scrubber contains *allicin,* an active sulfur-containing compound that is digestively transformed into *diallyldisulfide.* This initiates a powerful internal scrubbing action that reduces the lipid (fat) levels in your blood and liver. This same substance works swiftly to break down the accumulated fats and prepare them for elimination.

Eat Garlic with Each Meal   One or two garlic cloves chewed thoroughly or chopped and added to your meal will send forth this powerful allicin into your system to create the vital unplugging of your arteries. Garlic then acts as a miracle guardian against cholesterol waste overload. It is a dynamically powerful cell-scrubber that uproots and casts out this toxic waste.

A Clove a Day Keeps Cholesterol Way-Way-Way Down

Paul B. was a heavy construction worker who craved solid meat meals. A problem here was his excessively high cholesterol readings. His company doctor prescribed the daily use of garlic, along with suggestions on some reduction of fat intake. Paul B. liked the tangy taste of garlic and would consume as many as four cloves either with or at the end of his lunch and dinner. His breakfast was usually light, so it needed no garlic cleanser. In nine days, Paul B.'s cholesterol levels dropped at least 30 milligrams. At the end of 14 days, he was told that he had a satisfactory level. He continued enjoying his favorite foods and the garlic "dessert" as he happily called it. But just one clove a day was enough to keep his cholesterol at a healthy level.

LECITHIN WASHES AWAY CHOLESTEROL SLUDGE

What Is It?   Lecithin is a bland, water-soluble, granular powder made from de-fatted soybeans. Biochemists call it a *phosphatide,* that is, an essential component of all living cells and tissues. It is a prime source of phosphorus and nitrogen.

How Does It Wash Sludge?   A digestive enzyme, *lecithinase,* takes ingested lecithin and promotes the release of its *choline* (a B-complex vitamin) into the bloodstream. This lecithin-released choline now is able to break down cholesterol deposits and actually wash them right out of your system. Lecithin also contains lipo-tropic agents which metabolize the sludge and bring about its elimination.

Special Cleanser: Lecithin contains substances which clear up vitreous opacities (a colorless thickening, the forerunner of choles-terol deposits) and wash them out of your cells before they are able to accumulate to sludge-like levels.

Breaks Down Fatty Wastes   Lecithin boosts the distribution of *esterases* (enzyme activators) in the bloodstream, which act swiftly to break down fatty waste accumulations and provide you with clean arteries and a healthier body, too.

Double-Action Cell Cleansing   Lecithin is a prime source of two cell cleansers: *phosphatides* and *sitosterols*. They have the unique power of breaking down plaques and preparing them for elimina-tion. This gives you double-action cell cleansing that works swiftly and effectively.

Melts, Eliminates Thick Cholesterol in Twelve Days

Susan O. was told by her cardiologist that she had unusually high levels of cholesterol. The problem was serious because the wastes were thick and resisted usual dietary methods of dissolution. Susan O. was told to take from six to eight tablespoons of lecithin granules daily (available at health stores). She could mix them with vegetable juices, or sprinkle over cereals, salads, in stews, soups, casseroles. Susan O. followed this advice, cutting down on animal fat foods, too. Within twelve days, the stubborn cholesterol plaques succumbed to the emulsifying power of the lecithin and actually washed right out of her body. Her cardiologist offered the good news that she had healthy cholesterol levels, thanks to the lecithin program.

PECTIN FOR BALANCE OF HDL-LDL REACTIONS

What Is It?   Pectin is a water-soluble substance in plant foods that yields a gel used as the basis for jellies. It is a natural cell-scrubber derived mainly from plant cell walls and citrus fruit pulp. Now, it has been found to possess the power of being able to balance the delicate HDL-LDL levels in your bloodstream.

HDL Versus LDL   These are two different substances that are poles apart. One causes wastes to accumulate. The other helps scrub them out. Let's see the difference.

1. HDL stands for *High-Density Lipoprotein*, a form of fat circulating in your bloodstream. But it is a beneficial type in the sense that it is a cleanser. The more HDLs you have, the cleaner your cells are.

2. LDL stands for *Low-Density Lipoprotein*, a form of cholesterol sludge that accumulates in your bloodstream. It has been noted that too-high levels of the LDL sludge cause a risk of arterial and coronary ill health.

Problem: In many situations, an excess of LDLs will "overpower" the HDLs. This causes the cells to become filled with fatty wastes and the health risk increases.

Why This Conflict? Because water and fat do not mix, your body needs a system for dislodging excess fatty wastes (including cholesterol) and transporting it through the medium of your bloodstream for excretion. Proteins are used for this purpose. Scientists have named the two major groups of cholesterol-protein aggregates HDLs and LDLs.

What's the Difference? Here is the key to solving this internal struggle. HDLs act like cell-scrubbers, moving throughout your body via your bloodstream, searching out plaques and wastes and removing them from your cells; then the scrubbing HDLs carry these wastes to your liver and other eliminative channels. That is a vital cleansing action

Opposing this action are the LDLs. These act as "delivery trucks" by picking up fats, wastes, cholesterol, toxic clumps, and actually depositing them throughout your cells, especially in your blood vessels.

What's the Danger? Your basic arterial-coronary and general health depends on the balance of this removal-delivery system. If you have an excess of the LDL levels, then your cells become overloaded, even overflowing with wastes and refuse. *The Answer:* Boost your release of the cleansing HDLs so that they are able to gather up these wastes and prepare them for elimination.

How Pectin Creates This Vital Balance   While the preceding super-foods are also instrumental in boosting your cell-scrubbing HDLs, the food that can exert a most powerful influence on maintaining a balance is pectin.

Boosts HDLs, Washes Cells   When pectin enters your metabolism, it works speedily in boosting levels of HDLs so that they can "attack" cholesterol and waste products and prevent an overload. Pectin boosts the vigor of HDLs so they can more effectively wash your cells.

Dynamic Power of Pectin   An indigestible fiber, pectin becomes converted to an acid that combines with cholesterol, triglycerides, and wastes, to form an insoluble salt. Then it eliminates this "package" of debris. Similarly, pectin binds with many of these plaque-like toxic wastes and blocks their absorption within your cells and both on and in your arteries. Pectin actually seizes these wastes and sends them through your eliminative channel. All this is done by boosting the helpful HDL levels so that the choking LDL levels are overcome.

How to Take Pectin   Be not deceived! Consuming big gobs of jelly is *not* the good way to get pectin. You'll only fill up on sugar (a toxic-causing, non-nutritive, so-called food), which comprises up to 75% of most jellies. You'll also be adding calories to your body, not to mention other ailments caused by sugar, so pass up that method. Instead, you will find pectin in apples. Whether whole, sliced, grated, or made into applesauce (without sugar or artificial ingredients), you'll have adequate amounts of pectin. Be sure to eat the skin (after washing the fruit, of course) where pectin exists in its highest concentration. *Tip:* One apple has about two grams of pectin. Ten grams daily are helpful in raising the cell-scrubbing HDL levels to guard against toxic waste overload.

Other sources of pectin include such fresh fruits as bananas, pineapples, cherries, grapes, peaches, raspberries, sun-dried raisins. Also try tomatoes, avocados, carob, sunflower seeds, sesame seeds. Plan to eat these foods daily in any desired combination. You'll be boosting your HDL levels and controlling the amount of sludge that the undesirable LDLs would otherwise be dumping on your cells.

THREE EASY WAYS TO BOOST CELL-WASHING
ACTIONS

Your goal is to block overreaction of LDLs and to increase the cell-washing functions of the HDLs. To do so, you will need to establish an internal ratio so that you have more HDLs. In addition to consuming pectin in your daily foods, you should follow these three ways to boost the cell-washing actions and improve your health, too.

1. *Give up smoking.* It knocks out the beneficial high-density lipoproteins. At the same time, it actually raises the cell-dirtying, low-density lipoproteins. To avoid this internal reaction, give up smoking. It's good for your total health, too.

2. *Keep physically active.* Regular exercise boosts your levels of important HDLs. You could try doctor-approved exercise, mild jogging, even regular walking. These physical activities boost these HDLs and simultaneously increase the cell-washing action. *Caution:* A sedentary lifestyle may boost sludge-depositing LDLs and this increases your risk of cardiovascular disorders. So keep active and you'll keep your cells clean.

3. *Make dietary adjustments.* Control caloric intake. Reduce animal fats. You would do well to substitute vegetable oils and fats for so-called hard fats as much as possible. *Tip:* Fish contains the beneficial polyunsaturated fatty acids that boost HDLs and increase cellular cleanliness. Also, include garlic, brewer's yeast, and lecithin in your daily meal plan. They are powerful boosters for your cell-washing, high-density lipoproteins.

Exchanges "Old Body" for "New Body" in 30 Days

Adele Y. complained of chronic fatigue; her job as a store saleswoman required much standing and walking, and she found it increasingly difficult to wait on customers. Her face looked haggard. Her breath was short. She complained of stiff arms and joints. Adele Y. faced loss of her job and the threat of becoming an invalid. Complaining to her cardiologist, Adele Y. was examined and told that her basic problem was that of "arterial sludge." Not only did she have excessive cholesterol, but dangerously low levels of the important cell-washing, high-density lipoproteins. Immediately, she was put on a low animal fat program. She was also advised to take garlic, brewer's yeast, lecithin, and pectin daily. Adele Y. felt the improvement almost from the start. Energy increased. Her skin firmed up. She breathed easily and her limbs became flexible and she looked more vibrant. By the end of three weeks on this simple program, Adele Y. was as lively as a youngster. By the thirtieth day, she felt reborn and quipped that she had exchanged her old body for a new body . . . and she looked it, too! All this, thanks to the cell-scrubbing power of the miracle foods and low animal fat program. Her cardiologist informed her, happily, that she had very satisfactory cholesterol levels, too.

TEN WAYS TO PROTECT AGAINST CHOLESTEROL OVERLOAD

Make some minor adjustments in your food program. You'll help protect yourself against overloading your cells with cholesterol sludge. Here's a set of suggestions for cleaning your organs . . . and keeping them clean.

1. Eat no more than three egg yolks a week, including those in cooking.

2. Limit your use of shellfish and organ meats.

3. In any planned meat meals for the week, use fish, poultry, and veal; limit beef or lamb to five moderate-sized portions per week.

4. Choose lean cuts of meat. Trim visible fat. Discard fat that cooks out of the meat.

5. Avoid deep fat frying; use cooking methods that help remove fat—baking, boiling, broiling, roasting, stewing.

6. Restrict (better yet, avoid) use of fatty luncheon and variety meats such as sausages, salami, etc.

7. Instead of butter and other solid or hydrogenated fats, use liquid vegetable oils that are rich in waste-washing polyunsaturates.

8. Instead of whole milk products, use those made from low-fat or fat-free milk.

9. Egg whites do not contain cholesterol so you can eat them regularly. They also contain lecithin, a powerful sludge-washer, so this can be a power food for your program.

10. Daily, consume at least three or four cloves of garlic. This

miracle food not only lowers cholesterol, but also shrinks the most harmful part of that fat—the low-density lipoprotein (LDL) fraction. *Bonus:* Garlic reduces the tendency of blood platelets to clump together abnormally because of weighty toxic wastes. Such a clumping can predispose a threatening blood clot (forerunner of stroke or heart attack or both!). So be sure to wash your cells with the intake of garlic every single day!

YOUR CHOLESTEROL-WATCHING CHART

As explained above, cholesterol is found in foods and also is made by your body. So you would do well to control intake of this substance because an excess can easily occur if you take in more than about 300 to 400 milligrams daily.

Here's a chart listing common foods and their cholesterol content. Plan your meals with proper levels in mind daily. You'll help keep your body clean and make it easier for the power foods to control HDL-LDL levels, the key to internal washing.

CHOLESTEROL

Elevated blood cholesterol has been identified as one of the major factors associated with an increased risk of developing coronary heart disease.

Cholesterol is an essential fat-like substance found in all body cells. Our bodies manufacture cholesterol out of materials derived from foods we eat.

By lowering the intake of both *dietary cholesterol* and of *saturated fats*, blood cholesterol can be lowered.

Cholesterol is present in animal food products—meats, poultry, fish, eggs, and dairy products containing butter fat. Common foods highest in cholesterol are brains, kidney, sweetbreads, liver, and egg yolk.

Cholesterol is not found in plant foods—fruits, vegetables, grain and cereal products or nuts.

PRINCIPAL SOURCES OF CHOLESTEROL

Food and Description	Edible Amount	Milligrams Cholesterol
Eggs		
Chicken, whole	1 large	274
Chicken, white only	1 large	0
Duck, whole	1 large	619
Organ Meats		
Brains, beef, calf, pork, lamb	3½-oz. raw	1985
Heart, beef	3½-oz. cooked	274

PRINCIPAL SOURCES OF CHOLESTEROL

Food and Description	Edible Amount	Milligrams Cholesterol
Heart, chicken	3½-oz. cooked	231
Kidney, beef, calf, pork, lamb	3½-oz. cooked	804
Liver, beef, calf, pork, lamb	3½-oz. cooked	438
Liver, chicken	3½-oz. cooked	746
Sweetbreads	3½-oz. cooked	466
Meat		
Beef, bone removed	3½-oz. cooked	94
Chicken, flesh and skin—breast	3½-oz. cooked	80
Chicken, flesh and skin—drumstick	3½-oz. cooked	91
Lamb, bone removed	3½-oz. cooked	98
Pork, bone removed	3½-oz. cooked	89
Turkey, flesh and skin	3½-oz. cooked	93
Veal, bone removed	3½-oz. cooked	101
Shellfish		
Clams, soft	12 large raw	72
Crabs, steamed in shell	1 cup meat	125
Crabs, canned	½-cup packed	80
Lobster, cooked	1 cup meat	123
Oysters, Eastern	12 raw	90
Shrimp, canned drained solids	½-cup	96
	(approx. 12 large)	
Fish		
Cod, flesh only	3½-oz. raw	50
Cod, dried, salted	3½-oz.	82
Flounder, flesh only	3½-oz. raw	50
Haddock, flesh only	3½-oz. raw	60
Halibut, flesh only	3½-oz. raw	50
Herring, flesh only	3½-oz. raw	85
Herring, canned, solids and liquids	3½-oz.	97
Mackerel, flesh only	3½-oz. raw	95
Mackerel, canned, solids and liquids	3½-oz.	95
Roe, salmon	1 oz. raw	101
Salmon, sockeye or red—flesh only	3½-oz. raw	35
Salmon, canned, solids and liquids	3½-oz.	35
Sardines, canned in oil, drained solids	3½-oz.	140
Tuna, canned in oil, drained solids	3½-oz.	65
Fats		
Butter, regular	1 Tbsp.	33
Butter, whipped	1 Tbsp.	22
Cream, heavy	1 Tbsp.	21
Cream, light	1 Tbsp.	10
Cream, half and half	1 Tbsp.	6
Cream, sour	1 Tbsp.	5

PRINCIPAL SOURCES OF CHOLESTEROL

Food and Description	Edible Amount	Milligrams Cholesterol
Lard	1 Tbsp.	13
Margarine, all vegetable fat	1 Tbsp.	0
Mayonnaise	1 Tbsp.	10
Milk and Milk Products		
Cheese, cheddar	1 oz.	30
Cheese, processed American	1 oz.	27
Cheese, cottage, creamed	½-cup	16
Cheese, cottage, low fat (2% fat)	½-cup	10
Cheese, cream	1 oz.	31
Cheese, ricotta, whole milk	½-cup	63
Cheese, ricotta, partially skim milk	½-cup	38
Ice Cream, regular (approx. 10% fat)	1 cup	59
Ice Cream, rich (approx. 16% fat)	1 cup	88
Ice Cream, French, soft serve	1 cup	153
Ice Cream, frozen custard	1 cup	97
Ice Milk, hardened	1 cup	18
Ice Milk, soft serve	1 cup	13
Milk, whole	1 cup	33
Milk, low fat, 2% fat	1 cup	19
Milk, low fat, 1% fat	1 cup	10
Milk, nonfat (skim)	1 cup	5
Milk, chocolate flavored milk	1 cup	30
Milk, buttermilk, cultured	1 cup	9
Yogurt, whole milk, plain	1 cup	29
Yogurt, lowfat, plain	1 cup	14
Yogurt, lowfat, fruit varieties	1 cup	12
Yogurt, skim milk, plain	1 cup	4

WRAP-UP

1. Cholesterol overload = internal sludge. Control its intake and you will be rewarded with a more vigorous and youthful body and mind.

2. Paul B. used just a few garlic cloves to help "unplug" his sludge-covered arteries. Garlic acted as a miracle food in cleansing his body.

3. Susan O. was able to melt and eliminate thick clumps of cholesterol with the use of an all-natural food, lecithin. It worked wonders within twelve days.

4. The key to fat control lies in a balance of HDL-LDL reac-

tions. It is pectin, found in everyday foods, that helps bring about this crucial, often lifesaving balance.

5. Raise beneficial HDLs by following the three easy cell-washing steps as outlined.

6. Adele Y. swapped an "old" body for a "new" one within 30 days on an easy artery-washing program.

7. Protect against cholesterol sludge overload with the suggestions found in this chapter.

8. Plan cholesterol intake with the use of the chart. Limit yourself to 300 to 400 milligrams daily.

CHAPTER 3

"Forever Young" Skin Through Catalytic Cleansing

You can smooth out wrinkles, clear up blemishes, and restore the glow of youth to your skin. Often, this delightful, fresh-faced look can occur within a few days. Through the simple method of catalytic cleansing, you get to the root cause of your so-called "aging" skin—namely, toxic wastes, which lie directly beneath your visible skin surface. Accumulated, they block the free passage of nutrition and aeration, thereby causing a "choked" stagnation that is seen in the form of deep furrows and stubborn blemishes. To better understand how simple home programs can give you a "forever young" skin, let's look at the problem and the internal washing solution.

PROBLEM—SKIN-AGING CELLULITE

What Is It?   Cellulite is a term that was coined in European health spas to describe those unsightly deposits that are most visible on thighs and buttocks and seem to stubbornly resist most exercises. Pronounced "cell-u-leet," these "hard-to-budge pudge" bulges also accumulate just beneath the skin in the upper arms, back of the neck, shoulders, throat, and the face, too.

What Does It Look Like?   Cellulite is composed of lumpy deposits that resemble chicken skin or a puckery orange skin. Often, it is called the "orange rind" problem. You can *see* cellulite in the form of unattractive bulges, wrinkles, and creases as well as blemishes and discolorations.

What Is the Cause?   Certain body cells have the capacity to store huge amounts of fat; about half of your body's fat is deposited in these cells immediately beneath your skin. Strands of fibrous tissues connect the skin to deeper tissue layers, and also separate the fat cell compartments. When the fat cells increase in size, this simultaneously causes the compartments of fat to bulge and produce a "waffled" appearance on your skin, similar to the pattern of irregularities on the surface of an orange. *Quick Self-Test:* Compress a skin fold lightly between your fingers. See those imperfections? That's the penalty of cellulite.

Is Waste Accumulation a Factor?   Waste accumulation is perhaps the sole factor in the development of cellulite, which is a consequence of "fat-gone-wrong." That is, a combination of fat, water, and toxic wastes that ordinarily should be eliminated from your body but still remains and even accumulates.

Why Is This Fat-Waste Sludge Difficult to Remove?   Unlike other sludge accumulations, these wastes gather in the connective tissues that hold fat cells just beneath the skin's surface. Here, round fat cell chambers are found, along with thin epidermis and corium (outer leaves), which become thinner and less elastic in a person after the age of 30 and upward. These connective tissues harden and combine with the fat and water. Soon, there is formation of pockets of a gel-like substance that we call cellulite. A stubborn substance, it defies ordinary waste removal efforts and gives rise to skin aging that worsens as the years go on.

How Is Cellulite More Resistant Than Ordinary Fatty Deposits?   Cellulite contains more water and wastes than ordinary fatty tissue. The big problem is that gel-like cellulite tissue is *stagnant.* Locked, or worse, *trapped* in the cell chambers and the hardening epidermis-corium layers, the wastes cause unsightly bulges and skin blemishes, and appears to resist ordinary waste removal methods.

What Is the Biological Reason for Cellulite Formation?   The connective tissues and fat cells are allowed to accumulate wastes because there is a sluggishness on the part of the body's circulatory system, as well as the liver, which needs to filter toxins out of the cells. With the arrival of the age bracket of the 30s, there is a slight slowdown of the metabolic process. The reduction of the enzymatic cleansing method also allows wastes to cling together, to form this unsightly condition. It is considered a "penalty" of going into the middle years.

What Can Be Done to Improve Waste Removal Methods?   A set of home programs that wake up your sluggish metabolism helps. These programs are aimed at activating your glands and organs so that they promote more effective removal of wastes. The programs consist of both internal and external methods. In many situations the internal washing methods are so effective you can see results in a healthier skin in a matter of days, sometimes overnight.

FREE YOUR BODY OF CELLULITE IN SIX STEPS

Your goal is to dislodge the wastes that have formed a gelatin-like hardness in your connective tissues. You can set off an internal washing reaction by following this simple six-step cellulite-cleansing program right at home.

1. Foods That Fight Cellulite   Daily, boost your intake of fresh fruits and vegetables, lots of whole grain foods, limited amounts of meat (avoid fats), skim milk dairy products, and lots of fresh juices. *Avoid:* sugar, salt, caffeine, artificial foods, chemicals in foods, synthetics, preservatives, additives.

Catalytic Cleansing Benefit: Powerful enzymes found in raw fresh foods will work vigorously to dislodge and break up the clumps of fat-waste accumulations. These enzymes initiate a catalytic cleansing reaction that propels cellulite wastes right out of your eliminative channels. *Special Reward:* By eliminating the foods above you free your body from the onslaught of more wastes. This makes the catalytic removal of wastes all the easier and swifter, too.

2. Clean Insides = Youthful Outsides   Establish regularity by eating high-roughage foods such as wheat germ, bran, whole grains, fresh fruits and vegetables daily. Once you are "regular," your wastes are removed speedily. This is a simple way of washing out your overclogged cells and tissues.

Catalytic Cleansing Benefit: Cellulite is an internal clogging problem; therefore, when you consume these high-roughage and fiber foods you stimulate your sluggish metabolism into more vigorous action. Elimination becomes more complete. You remove cellular wastes and help overcome the problem of those unsightly bulges.

3. Breathe Away Toxic Wastes   Your choked cells need oxygen. Deprived of this "breath of life," they tend to weaken. Clinging together, they also start to harden because they lack nutrients transported via the oxygenation process. Without the free exchange of air and carbon dioxide, the cells "choke" and become stagnant. They accumulate wastes and the cellulite syndrome develops. Daily, deep-breathe your way to cellular washing. In the open air or before an open window (avoid drafts or chills) stand and inhale deeply; hold it for the count of five. Exhale all the way. Repeat 10 to 15 times each morning. Repeat at night.

Catalytic Cleansing Benefit: The gentle forceful intake of oxygen will transport needed nutrients to your waste-burdened cells and tissues. Invigorated, your cells now begin the metabolic process of uprooting and casting out toxic wastes. Give your cells the "breath of life." Clean them through simple inhalation exercises daily. Increase your circulation. Invigorated cells are cellulite-free cells.

4. Massage Away Those Unsightly Bulges   A miracle rub is possible with the use of a loofah "sponge," available at most health stores and pharmacies as well as beauty supply outlets. The loofah (it grows like a gourd) is a member of the cucumber family. It is fibrous—more than an ordinary massage item. Thousands of these little "needles" rubbed over the bulgy area will dislodge wastes and prepare them for elimination. Use the loofah wet or dry. Loofahs are also available as a hand mitt for easy self-rubbing. Just rub all over your body for about 20 minutes daily, preferably after a bath, and you will soon be rewarded in terms of a smoother skin.

Catalytic Cleansing Benefit: A loofah will cleanse and stimulate your skin surface. The steady friction penetrates deeper into the lower skin layers, and tends to break down and eventually disintegrate accumulated fats and wastes. Stroke the area briskly (but not roughly) in the direction of your heart. Performed daily, this promotes a rhythmic removal of cellulite wastes.

5. Keep Your Body in Tiptop Shape   Simple exercises such as deep knee bends, ordinary walking, and doctor-approved jogging, help keep your circulation boosted. A more vigorous metabolic reaction will help maintain improved cell washing so that wastes are not allowed to accumulate. Plan to do simple exercises for 30 minutes each day. You'll be giving your body the vigor required for cellulite cleansing.

   Catalytic Cleansing Benefit: Stagnation needs corrective movement. When you exercise, you set off a chain reaction which signals your body processes to boost metabolic flushing out of fats and wastes. You also trigger off a more improved caloric burning reaction that ignites and actually causes a spontaneous combustion reaction upon dissolved wastes. This makes elimination more effective. Keep your body in tiptop active condition. You'll look and feel much younger.

6. Relax Away Those Accumulated Wastes   Tension, unrelieved stress, pent-up emotions are often responsible for waste buildup. The cause is traced to a "choked up" emotional-physical situation. This tightness is reflected in clumped-up wastes that lead to skin problems and related disorders. *Example:* You can feel the penalties of tension when you are so much under stress that you become constipated! This suggests a change in attitude and lifestyle. Plan to have more recreation. Wherever possible, avoid disputes. Shield yourself from excessive responsibilities. Take frequent rest breaks and relax yourself. In so doing, you improve your body's ability to wash away locked-up wastes.

   Catalytic Cleansing Benefit: Loosened-up muscles will help release "kinks" in your arteries, veins, circulatory system, and vital organs. Once these channels are opened up, there is a freer exchange of oxygen and nutrients. Catalytic hormones are able to bring about a more effective dissolution of stubborn clumps and then eject them from your body. By "unlocking" your tension-caused "blockages," you are able to rid yourself of unattractive cellulite.

Works Swiftly, Effectively, Permanently, Too   The preceding easy-to-follow cellulite-freedom program works swiftly. The six steps are effective in restoring better metabolism so that you may be permanently rid of cellulite, the cause of older-looking skin.

Becomes "Forever Young" in One Weekend

Joyce N. was so embarrassed by her wrinkled, furrowed skin she wore long-sleeved garments, high-necked dresses, and wide-brimmed hats to cover her puckered forehead. Costly cosmetics just disguised the problem which was identified as cellulite by a dermatologist. Joyce N. was told she could wash out her cellulite with the preceding six-step program, which would revive her sluggish metabolism. It would create a catalytic action so that stubborn fats and wastes could be dislodged and eliminated. Joyce N. followed the program over a long weekend. Within three days, her wrinkles "ironed out." Her furrows smoothed. Her entire skin was silky soft and rose-colored again. She smilingly boasted she was now "forever young" with just one weekend on this six-step program.

CATALYTIC SKIN CLEANSERS FOR COMMON AND UNCOMMON DISORDERS[1]

Cleanse away skin disorders with these at-home programs, which are aimed at opening pores, creating a catalytic cleansing action, and strengthening your cells so that they are firm, youthful, healthy. Many of these programs work after one or two applications; some require a bit more time. Proceed at your own pace. You have nothing to lose . . . except your aging, blemished skin!

Acne. Apply thin slices of fresh cucumber on acne-plagued areas for 15 minutes. Remove slices. Splash with cold water. Pat dry. Repeat three times daily.

Dry Skin. Wash your face with a mild soap and warm water. Separate an egg and beat the yolk. Apply to your face. Let yolk harden. After 20 minutes, splash off with warm and cool water. Repeat several times daily. (Remember to keep egg white for use in cooking.)

Oily Skin. With finger tips, apply plain yogurt to oily areas. Let yogurt remain for 20 minutes. Splash off with tepid water. Repeat several times daily.

---

[1]*Natural Health Bulletin,* Delta Group, 1101D State Road, Princeton, N.J. 08540. Selected issues from years 1979 through 1981. Available by subscription.

Tired Skin. In your palm, combine oatmeal with enough water to make a grainy paste. Gently rub your face with this grainy mixture until dry skin flakes off. Finish with a cold water splash.

Neck Wrinkles. Dip a clean face towel in warm olive oil. Wrap towel around your throat. Cover with a dry towel. After 30 minutes, remove towels and shower off any oil residue. This helps moisturize your neck, steam away toxic wastes, and guard against wrinkles.

Puffy Eyes. Dip cotton balls in milk; apply to your closed eyes. Lie down for 20 minutes. Remove pads and splash with cool water.

Pineapple Skin Cleanser. Into ¼ cup pineapple juice, dip thick gauze and apply gently to blemished areas of your skin. Let juice remain for 20 minutes, then rinse with tepid water. Repeat twice daily. *Benefits:* Pineapple enzymes help remove the top layer of dead skin cells and improve tissue regeneration.

Grape Juice Rinse. Dip clean gauze into a bowl of grape juice. Rub all over your face. Let remain for five minutes. Rinse with tepid and cool water. *Benefits:* The tart elements of the grape juice will penetrate skin pores and promote cleansing and subsequent cellular regeneration.

Watermelon Pack. Blenderize and strain pitted watermelon chunks. Wrap the pulp in cheesecloth to form a facial pack. Apply this pack to your face. Let remain for 20 minutes. Splash off with cool water. Repeat several times daily. *Benefits:* Nutrients and enzymes in the pack cleanse your pores and provide moisture. Watermelon juice helps quench "thirsty" cells beneath skin surface and protects against wrinkles.

Berry Mask. Wash and hull a handful of strawberries. Mash with a wooden spoon until smooth. Apply berry mixture to blemishes. Let dry for 20 minutes. Then splash off with tepid water. *Benefits:* The high enzyme content catalyzes toxic wastes, promotes cleansing, creates a glowing skin.

Peachy Complexion. Pit and blenderize several ripe peaches. Smooth on your face as you would a skin cream; it is preferable to leave on overnight. *Benefits:* Peach minerals seep through delicate pores and membranes to promote internal washing and a more youthful skin.

Dry Skin. Try a moisturizing or hydrotherapy treatment. Fill tub with warm, *not* hot water (which is drying to the skin). Add one-half cup of ordinary vegetable oil. Soak comfortably while gently washing your face and body with a soft cloth for no more than 15 minutes. Dry with a soft towel, but do not rub. Remember, dry skin is delicate, so treat it with kindness and it will moisturize more effectively.

Deep Lines, Creases. Give yourself a gentle massage. Dip fingertips into vegetable oil. Gently massage into the dry portions of your face, always *away* from the direction in which lines tend to form. *Suggestion:* Use an up-and-away motion. Begin at the base of your throat, then work upward and finish at your temples. Let the thin film of oil remain overnight to further moisturize and cleanse while you sleep. Next morning, splash it off with warm and cool water. After a few days, your skin will start to smooth out.

Aging Furrows. Mix one handful of raw oatmeal with enough hot mineral water to form a paste; spread onto your face and throat. After it has dried, let remain on your face for 30 minutes. Rinse with cool mineral water. Watch your creases and wrinkles just "melt" away.

Blackheads, Pitted Dirt. Combine a teaspoon of almond meal (from health store) with enough mineral water to form a creamy lotion. Moisten face and throat with mineral water; now rub this almond mixture gently into your skin with the finger tips. Let dry. Splash off with cool water. Used daily, it helps get rid of blackheads and smooths out those pitted dirt-filled pores.

Pore Cleanser and Refiner. Add a pinch of powdered alum (from health store or pharmacy) to enough hot water to form a thin solution. Pat on unsightly pores. When dry, splash off with cool water. This cleanses and then tightens enlarged pores and helps to refine skin.

Total Body Cleanser. Just add some dry milk to your bathwater. Soak yourself in this milk bath and luxuriate for 30 minutes. You'll emerge with a clean body that will look and feel younger.

Rub Away Those Blemishes. Try peels of citrus fruits on blemishes. Orange rind is a helpful complexion softener and facial massage. Grapefruit or lemon peel rubs away chapped blemishes. Just rub on affected area gently, as often as possible. Blemishes will begin to clear up almost from the start.

Flaking Skin. Combine one tomato with enough buttermilk to make a smooth paste. Spread over your face, rubbing gently. Let remain for 30 minutes. Splash off with warm and cool water. Wastes and decaying cells are sloughed off. You'll emerge with a smoother skin.

Enlarged Pores. Beat one egg white with one teaspoon of lemon juice until stiff. Apply to enlarged pores and blemishes. Let remain for 30 minutes. Wash off with cool water. Pores will start to tighten almost at once.

Overnight Skin Cleanser. Combine one tablespoon butter, two tablespoons honey and one egg yolk. Blend until creamy. Apply to face overnight. It works with catalytic cleansing action *while you sleep.* Next morning, splash off with warm and cool water. Discover a brand new and youthful face smiling happily at you in the mirror.

Steam Away Blemishes. Fill a washbowl with hot water. Toss in a handful of your favorite herbs. Now cover your head with a cloth, making a tent. Steam-open your pores for 20 to 30 minutes. The herbal scents will penetrate into your open pores and help promote a fragrant cleansing. Now, just splash off with cool water to close pores. Blemishes will be cleansed away after a few home steam treatments.

CATALYTIC CLEANSING—BABY SKIN
AT ANY AGE

You can enjoy a skin that is forever young with the use of these catalytic cleansing programs. When you uproot, loosen, dissolve, and wash away toxic debris, you regenerate your skin cells. When cleansed and nourished, they give more youthful support to your body envelope—your skin. Result? You have a baby-smooth skin, at any age. You do deserve the best that nature has to offer. Take it and de-age your skin and entire body.

IN REVIEW

1. To have a "forever young" skin, try catalytic cleansing of cellulite, the underlying cause of visible aging.

2. Just six simple steps, built into your daily lifestyle, will help free your body of cellulite.

3. Joyce N. was able to erase her wrinkles and become young again in just one weekend on a simple program.

4. Find your skin problem and the proper catalytic cleansing remedy.

CHAPTER

4

How to Balance Your Blood Pressure with Internal Washing

High blood pressure (hypertension) is a reaction to the accumulation of wastes that are "bursting at the seams" to be eliminated. These toxins play havoc with your pressure, causing distressing and often dangerous irregularities. To understand how wastes create this imbalance and how internal washing can restore normal levels, let's understand the basics about this situation.

WHAT DOES "BLOOD PRESSURE" MEAN?

Blood pressure refers to the amount of force exerted in the bloodstream as it passes through the arteries. When the left ventricle of your heart contracts, or squeezes down, it forces your blood out into the arteries. The major arteries then expand to receive the oncoming blood.

How Pressure Occurs The muscular linings of your arteries resist the pressure; the blood is squeezed out into the smaller vessels of your body. Blood pressure is the combined amount of pressure the blood is under as a result of the pumping of the heart, the resistance of the arterial walls, and the closing of the heart valves.

How Is Blood Pressure Diagnosed? There are two basic terms involved:

1. *Systolic Pressure.* The pressure at which your heart pumps blood into your arteries—the top figure in a diagnostic reading.

2. *Diastolic Pressure.* This is the minimum pressure, which exists when your heart is at peak relaxation; or, the pressure in your arteries *between* heartbeats. This is the bottom figure in a diagnostic reading.

What Is a Normal Level?   A systolic/diastolic reading of "120 over 80" is considered normal.

What Are Risky Levels?

Borderline Hypertension—A reading of 140/90.

Mild Hypertension—A reading of 170/105.

Moderate Hypertension—A reading of 185/115.

Severe Hypertension—A reading of 220/140 *and over.*

BEWARE PROLONGED HYPERTENSION

Everyone needs blood pressure. It moves blood through your circulatory system. Pressure goes up and down within a limited range. But when this pressure goes up and *stays up,* it creates hypertension. This places your heart and arteries under an abnormal amount of strain. The excess pressure constantly pounds all body organs nourished by the blood supply. Prolonged high blood pressure worsens any heart condition, forces the heart to work harder, and also accelerates the process of atherosclerosis.

More Risks: A blood vessel in the brain may burst, causing a stroke. There is impairment of the kidneys' ability to filter out wastes, thus causing toxic buildup. The heart, which must work harder to pump blood against the increased pressure in the arteries, may begin to show signs of strain. If ignored, high blood pressure can cause irreversible body injury.

Hypertensives have four times more heart attacks than those with normal blood pressure. And when a hypertensive does fall victim to such a heart attack, it is much more likely to be fatal.

TOXIC WASTE OVERLOAD—ROOT CAUSE OF RUNAWAY BLOOD PRESSURE

The accumulation of toxic wastes is a key factor in erratic and runaway readings of blood pressure. Consuming synthetics; salt residue; artificial ingredients; excessive fat; and irritating stimulants such as coffee, tea, soft drinks, all cause the deposition of these toxic wastes on the vital segments of your cardiovascular system.

Toxins Cause Risky Pressure Rise   Accumulation of these wastes creates deposits that stick to the walls of your arteries. Glue-like, these toxins narrow the channels through which blood and oxygen must travel to nourish your body. This condition still allows your heart and arteries to perform, but it ultimately adds to the risk of causing what doctors label as "congestive heart failure." To guard against this threat to your health, your goal should be the internal washing of these sludge deposits on your arteries. When cleansed, you can then balance your blood pressure and enjoy a more vigorous, youthful lifestyle.

GARLIC WASHES YOUR ARTERIES, BALANCES YOUR BLOOD PRESSURE

This miracle, lifesaving food has the power to uproot and dislodge the artery-choking sludge deposits and cast them out of your body. This paves the way for a balanced blood pressure.

Cleans Arteries   When additional garlic is included in your food program, it is able to dissolve a harmful toxic waste that sticks to your low-density lipoprotein (LDL) factor. Garlic, because of its allicin content, is able to scrub away the toxic wastes and cleanse arteries so there is a better distribution of blood carrying oxygen. By opening up arterial channels, there is a corresponding relief from forced blood pumping, thus the pressure is restored to a normal reading. Just include garlic daily for this internal washing benefit.

Washes Clot Risk   In toxic overload, the glue-like wastes actually cause blood platelets to clump together. This platelet sludge can lead to a dangerous blood clot. But garlic is able to wash away the gluey substance and protect against that tendency. Once the sludge is cleansed, the mobile platelets are liberated and do not present the risk of a clot. Again, by eating garlic daily, you can wash away this blood clot risk.

Improves Basic Circulation   A unique benefit of garlic is in its power to increase what is called *fibrinolyctic activity*. It exerts its allicin power as well as its mitogenetic radiation factor, which stimulates the flow of blood. This causes your fibrins (protein-like substances) to become cleansed and thereby become free of the sludge that would choke off circulation and predispose a risk of clotting. Clean fibrins = clean circulation, which also means a balanced blood pressure. This is possible with the use of circulation-cleansing garlic.

GARLIC + ONIONS = HEALTHY BLOOD PRESSURE

A combination of these two special vegetables can work miracles in providing you with a healthy blood pressure and a longer life, too.

Unique Power: Used in combination, both vegetables are able to (1) lower high levels of blood fats and, (2) reduce levels of fibrin, the substance that becomes filled with wastes and may cause blood clotting.

Powerful Substance Is Super-Cell Cleanser   In particular, onions contain a cell cleanser known as prostaglandin A1. When you eat onions together with garlic, this super-cell cleanser is doubly invigorated (more than if onions are eaten alone) and works swiftly to cause this fibrin-washing and lifesaving action.

Controls Dangerous Sludge   Garlic and onions (both members of the allium family) are able to control formation of a dangerous sludge known as *thromboxane*. This toxic waste causes platelet aggregation (clumping together). When this happens, pressure soars and a blood clot risk may be imminent. But eating garlic and onions daily will provide a buffering reaction to this threat. An even more vital benefit is that these miracle foods will wash away the thromboxane sludge and give you free-moving platelets . . . and a safe, sane, and healthy blood pressure level.

Plan to eat garlic daily, either chewed in clove form, or chopped fine and added to soups, stews, salads, casseroles, and baked foods of almost all varieties. You will be fortifying your metabolic system with the super-cleanser that will give you protection against sludge buildup and freedom from the risk of a fatal heart attack.

"Dangerous" Pressure Drops Overnight

Kate H. was told by her cardiovascular specialist that she had a blood pressure reading of 230/150. This was so dangerous, she was given a 50-50 chance of survival! Medications made her dizzy and nauseous. She needed help swiftly. The doctor advised her to consume at least one whole garlic daily (either raw or cooked in any desired way) together with several onions for better assimilation. Kate H. followed this program. Overnight, the miracle combination actually "devoured" the sludge that was choking her arterioles and eliminated them just as speedily. Next day, Kate H. went in for another reading. The specialist told her happily that it had dropped to 150/95—almost normal. Kate H. felt she had been snatched from the jaws of hypertension-caused heart failure by the scrubbing action of garlic and onions.

THE LOW-SALT WAY TO WASTE-FREE ARTERIES AND NORMAL PRESSURE

Salt from the shaker or as it appears in processed foods is a major cause of toxic sludge in your bloodstream. Certain substances in your blood become "coated" with salt residue. An excess of these cellular coatings can cause a stagnation that is the forerunner of high blood pressure.

Toxic Waste Reaction of Salt   When you consume salt, it encrusts your millions of cells. In this form, it builds up toxic wastes that narrow the passageways of your small arteries. This same waste will "choke" the glands so that there is a hormonal reduction, which also plays havoc with your blood pressure, as well as your general health. Salt wastes also tend to cause enlargement of the heart. This overload is more than just a cause of hypertension; it is a cause of premature death!

Sneaky Reaction of Salt-Wastes   When salt wastes are allowed to increase, they create a hydraulic effect by blocking vital fluids in your circulatory system. This causes blood pressure to zoom to an unhealthy and dangerous high. *Caution:* Salt intake for just a brief period of time (as minimal as one day) can induce sludge overload and hypertension from the start.

"Restored to Life" on a "Glue-Free" Food Program

As a technician, Philip T. was under much business pressure, which he thought contributed to his escalating blood pressure. But his company physician said that his intake of excessive amounts of salt compounds had caused "glue-like compounds" to "lock" his platelets together, choking off free blood circulation. Philip T. had a dangerously high reading of 260/150 that kept climbing. He was told if it went higher, it could be fatal! Swift action was needed to save his rapidly deteriorating condition. He eliminated all forms of salt and/or sodium. He switched to flavorful herbs and spices. Within nine days, his pressure dropped to a healthful 130/80. In effect, he had been "restored to life" on this "glue-free" program that now keeps him alive and happy. Stress had little to do with his near brush to death. Glue-forming foods did!

SIX WAYS TO MAINTAIN CLEAN ARTERIES AND BALANCED BLOOD PRESSURE

Sludge accumulation increases your risk of high blood pressure. But a few simple changes in your way of life (and eating) can help wash out this sludge and keep it out so that you can balance your blood pressure with clean arteries. The changes are easy to follow, and lifesaving, too.

1. *Avoid Salt Sediment.* Do not have this cause of toxic waste in your home. Avoid its use in foods. Read labels of packaged foods and be guided accordingly. Remember, use flavorful herbs and spices to give you the taste of sodium without its waste-causing penalties.

2. *Boost Potassium Intake.* This mineral is an effective "blood washer" because it is able to boost your catalytic response; that is, it activates "messages" through your nervous system to send forth enzymes that help dilute and wash wastes out of your system. Eat high-potassium and low-sodium foods. They wash out blockages that otherwise raise blood pressure.

3. *Be Cautious About Hard Fats.* Animal fats (saturated) cling to your vital organs and choke off free transportation of blood and oxygen. Use them moderately, if at all. Switch to polyunsaturated oils, which have valuable essential fatty acids that break up and help wash away wastes.

4. *Unlock Blockage on Caffeine-Free Program*. Coffee, tea, chocolate products, and many "cola" beverages contain high concentrations of caffeine. This drug-like substance distorts your nervous system, "chokes" your circulation, and deposits sediment at crucial points. It also plays a role in hypertension. Switch to coffee substitutes, herbal teas, carob confections (but without sugar), and fresh juices. You will help unlock blockage and maintain a balanced blood pressure rhythm.

5. *Less Weight = Lower Blood Pressure*. Fat-encrusted cells and tissues cause excess weight as well as interference in the transport of nutrients. Lose that excess weight; wash out those burdensome fatty calories. This makes for a balanced level that enables your blood pressure to work more smoothly and efficiently.

6. *Exercise Away Toxic Wastes*. Physical activity, simple exercises, whatever helps pep up your sluggish system, will loosen up gathered toxic wastes and prepare them for elimination. Clinging wastes are "shaken free" with exercise and washed out of your body. Your blood can pump more efficiently without these blockages. You are rewarded with healthful blood pressure and freedom from the threat of hypertension.

Build these simple six steps into your lifestyle. You will be able to enjoy clean arteries and a satisfactory blood pressure level.

THE "SNACK" THAT CONTROLS BLOOD PRESSURE

Obey the urge to snack with garlic!

Carry a packet of garlic cloves in a tiny bottle. Chew thoroughly one clove to satisfy the snacking urge. You'll also be releasing a high concentration of a trace mineral called *selenium*. This mineral combines with garlic's biologically active anti-atherosclerotic ingredients to prevent platelet adhesion or clot blockage. Selenium is then activated by the garlic's ingredients to chip away and dissolve these adhesions or sediments and prepare them for expulsion.

Unusual Benefit: When garlic is consumed without other foods, its volatile actions are super-concentrated in force. It works more vigorously without interference in washing away cellular debris. It is better able to control blood pressure when consumed alone. So you can snack your way with powerful garlic to a balanced blood pressure.

Saves His Life with Simple Daily Snacks

"Either bring down that sky-high blood pressure, or get ready for a funeral . . . your own!" Those shocking words told Peter F. that his 375/220 reading could end his life at almost any moment. The problem was that this electrical engineer could not take medication. Its side effects ranged from falling asleep at the wheel or painful spasms. He needed swift treatment. He discussed the problem with an orthomolecular physician (nutrition-minded) who suggested he start snacking on garlic. He was to consume at least four whole garlic cloves daily, one at a time, of course. Immediately, the frightened Peter F. started chewing on the cloves. He boosted his intake to five whole garlic cloves daily "for good measure." In three days his reading dropped to 180/120. In five days, he had a reading of 125/80. His blockages had been dislodged and eliminated by the garlic ingredients. This miracle vegetable had saved his life, all with simple daily snacks!

WASH AWAY HYPERTENSION . . . WITHOUT DELAY

Hypertension is an ailment without symptoms, a "silent executioner." It is traced to toxic waste accumulations that prematurely age the body and strike down its victims with strokes, heart attacks, and/or kidney failure, often without much warning. That is why it is vital for you to nip hypertension in the bud . . . at the root cause of the problem, which calls for internal washing. But do it without delay!

High blood pressure is so symptomless that it is compared to a "time bomb" ticking away in your body. Don't wait until it goes off. Wash away that debris right now . . . while there is still time.

SUMMARY

1. Familiarize yourself with blood pressure and learn how internal cleansing can help save your life.
2. Garlic washes toxic wastes from your arteries and helps balance your pressure levels.
3. Garlic plus onions offer a double miracle in cleansing for speedy pressure control.

4. Kate H. dropped her "dangerous" pressure overnight on a simple tasty garlic plus onion program.

5. Avoid salt since it deposits sludge in your bloodstream to raise pressure. Note suggestions for salt watching and salt substituting.

6. Avoid the "glue-forming" compounds for balanced pressure.

7. This same "glue-free" program restored Philip I. to a new life with a healthier blood pressure.

8. A simple six-step program can wash away toxemia and improve pressure.

9. Use garlic as a snack to have around-the-clock protection. This method saved Peter F. from certain fatality with a skyrocketing blood pressure.

CHAPTER 5

How to Revitalize
Your Digestive System
for Total Youth

A sparklingly clean set of digestive organs is your key to total youth. These organs transform foods into nutrients that nourish and regenerate your body from head to toe. If these organs are clogged with wastes, their efficiency ratio is lowered. They cannot completely metabolize foods and so they become weak in their responsibility of assimilating youth-building elements. This may lead to general body decline and loss of vital responses. If the digestive organs become excessively saturated with glue-like wastes, premature aging begins and health starts to slip away, bit by bit. To protect yourself against this undesirable situation, your goal should be to cleanse away toxic wastes from your organs so they can perform smoothly and efficiently in helping you enjoy total youth.

HOW TO WASH AWAY THE "GLUE" THAT
CREATES CONSTIPATION

An accumulation of "glue-like" substances from improperly digested refined foods is often the cause of the blockage known as constipation. Your intestinal membranes become choked with artificial deposits from refined flour products as well as remnants of sugar and salt. These toxins clump together to create wedges that are barriers to the release of wastes.

61

POTASSIUM: THE MINERAL THAT OPENS UP TIGHT INTESTINAL ORGANS

Potassium is a waste-washing and organ-scrubbing mineral that opens up tight intestinal organs. It causes a gentle but effective contraction of the toxic-burdened sphincter muscles, a dislodging of the accumulated wastes.

Potassium further penetrates the intestinal cells and tissues of these muscles and alerts them to their organ-scrubbing responsibilities. Within moments, the stored-up contents are being readied for removal.

Sources of organ-scrubbing potassium are green leafy vegetables, oranges, whole grains, potatoes (especially the skin), bananas, apple cider vinegar, sun-dried apricots, figs, prunes.

THE 25¢ FRUIT THAT CAUSES SWIFT WASTE-WASHING

The humble-looking prune is a powerhouse of potassium, which causes swift waste-washing. Just a few prunes in the morning, at a cost of 25¢ or less, can create this organ-scrubbing action that will end the problem of constipation. Even more important, it's all done naturally!

How to Clean Your Digestive System in Minutes   In the morning, pour two cups of freshly boiled water over a few sun-dried prunes. In minutes, they will "plump" up and make it easier for you to remove the pits. When lukewarm, eat the prunes and then slowly sip the liquid. Do this on an empty stomach before breakfast.

Melts Glue, Unlocks Sludge, Removes Wastes   The high concentration of potassium works with Vitamin A (abundant in prunes) to stimulate the enzymatic process. This melts down the wastes, dissolves the blockages, and then propels them to eliminative channels. The lukewarm juice is a powerhouse of potassium and enzymes that further work to scrub away the intestines and free them of the toxic wastes that have become "pasted" together to cause constipation.

Corrects Lifelong Constipation in Three Days

Years of toxic waste overload made Dorothy P. feel miserable with her stubborn constipation. As a schoolteacher, she was sluggish in the morning when she had to be especially alert. Laxatives weakened her intestines, not to mention causing embarrassment at the most inconvenient times. She was constantly sluggish, had "sour stomach," and gas-like stomach rumbles. Dorothy P. had sallow, sagging skin. A sympathetic teacher suggested she consult a gastroenterologist. She was advised by this doctor to try the morning prune program. In just three days, it unblocked her channels. She was free from lifelong constipation . . . and for just 25¢ each morning! Her stomach was fresh and clean. Her skin became pink and firm. She felt reborn! She discovered that a "clean insides" will help create a "youthful outsides."

THE "MIRACLE SALAD" THAT REJUVENATES DIGESTIVE SYSTEM

The grime that clings stubbornly to digestive-eliminative organs is comparable to thick grease on a pipe. It grows in bulk until it covers the pipe and actually "chokes" its ability to function. So it is with your digestive organs. An overload or accumulation of toxic wastes will so clog up your vital organs, that your entire digestive-assimilative processes become weakened. This can lead to health-draining nutritional deficiencies that predispose one to the so-called aging process. This need not happen. With the use of a special "Miracle Salad" you can correct intestinal stagnation and give your vital organs a "full steam ahead" working pace. You will then enjoy total youth with total nutrition.

"Miracle Salad"—How It Promotes Swift Cleansing   Combine a few chopped garlic cloves with green leafy vegetables. Add a few slices of raw onion. Now sprinkle with just two or three tablespoons of apple cider vinegar and mix together. Eat this "Miracle Salad" *before* your main meal. If you wish, add some slices of natural cheese and a hard-boiled egg. Together with whole grain bread, it makes a complete meal in itself.

Benefits: The allicin substance in the garlic is invigorated by the minerals in the onion. In this combination, the allicin penetrates the large intestine along with the roughage of the raw green vegetables. The high potassium content of the apple cider vinegar boosts enzymatic action of the allicin. Now, this dynamic garlic substance stimulates the peristaltic movement of the sluggish and waste-covered intestinal walls. Almost at once, the allicin is able to dislodge the accumulated wastes and bring about swift cleansing.

A Salad a Day Keeps You Clean Forever   This simply prepared "Miracle Salad" can keep you clean forever if eaten daily, through the action of the dynamic garlic allicin compound. It's the all-natural way to actually dissolve accumulated toxic wastes and speedily eliminate them. Your body will then respond with more vigorous digestive action and improved assimilation of vital, youth-building nutrients.

How "Miracle Salad" Promoted "Total Youth" in Four Days

Internal sludge caused such intestinal blockage that Norah V. had a sallow look, felt tired even in mid-afternoon, was unable to relax, and developed unsightly sores all over her body. Her dermatologist wisely suggested they get to the root of her problem, which was intestinal blockage. The toxic wastes were releasing putrid fumes that caused cellular deterioration as well as collagen disintegration. To correct this problem, she needed speedy elimination of wastes. The doctor prescribed the "Miracle Salad" to be eaten after her noon meal, then again after her dinner. Norah V. followed the program hopefully. The first day, she felt long-awaited relief. The next day, she felt more energetic, and noticed that the blemishes were subsiding. The third day, her complexion became pink and smooth. She felt youthful vitality and at night she could enjoy refreshing sleep. The fourth day made her look rosy-cheeked and made her feel like a youngster again. The "Miracle Salad" had restored regularity and regenerated her powers of assimilation. Now she enjoyed "total youth," and it happened in four days.

Unplug Constipation with More Roughage   The sweeping action of enzyme-rich raw vegetables as well as whole grains (particularly wheat germ and bran) will unplug blockages and relieve constipation. Roughage will help revitalize your digestive system and give you the refreshing look and feel of youth . . . at any age.

HOW TO WASH AWAY THE IRRITANTS OF INDIGESTION

Indigestion refers to a group of symptoms that can be traced to toxic irritation caused by gastrointestinal blockage. You know you have indigestion by so-called heartburn or burning pain in your chest. You may even feel nauseated after just a few items of food or drink. It suggests that you need to wash away the irritants to enjoy a sparklingly clean digestive system.

Six Ways to End Problems of Indigestion   A few adjustments in your eating methods can control the intake of toxic wastes that lead to burning indigestion.

1. *Do not overeat.* Excessive indulgence causes your digestive enzymes to become overworked and not be able to break down food quickly. Decomposition of food occurs, which gives rise to toxic wastes and corroding fumes. Be moderate.

2. *Do not eat or drink too fast.* Gulped-down food that is improperly enzyme-digested will "rot" and give rise to digestive upset. Eat at a leisurely pace; drink slowly. Your digestive system is better able to accommodate these foods and will not protest.

3. *Do not swallow excessive air.* Called *aerophagia*, the gulping of air through the mouth while taking in food will upset the internal oxygenation of your system. This disturbs the enzymatic balance, and causes poor digestion, which leads to decomposed foods—the source of indigestion. Eating slowly and comfortably will reduce air intake.

4. *Chew your food thoroughly.* Doing so means that the enzymes in saliva prepare swallowed food for more complete digestion. Your digestive enzymes will be able to work more effectively on thoroughly chewed food. This avoids backup of chunks of decomposed and toxic-causing foods.

5. *Cook as thoroughly as required.* Undercooked food is difficult to digest, and may cause indigestion through the deposition of tough fibrous material. Make it a rule to cook certain foods thoroughly.

6. *Limit fat intake.* Animal fat is a major source of toxic waste accumulation. Because it is greasy, it tends to cling in clumps or droplets to the vital digestive (and body) organs. Since grease and water do not mix, such droplets remain resistant and tend to accumulate. Limit the intake of animal fats. Plan to complete a meal with a fresh raw fruit platter as dessert. The raw fruit enzymes are powerful and are able to wash away grease and help keep your digestive apparatus in a clean condition.

With these guidelines, you should be able to protect yourself against distressful indigestion.

HOW TO WASH AWAY THE PAIN OF ULCERS

An ulcer is a hole or an erosion in the tissue lining almost anywhere in the digestive tract. It is found most frequently in the duodenum or stomach. This crater-like sore in the thin membrane lining is caused by the corroding effect of accumulated wastes that stubbornly refuse to be washed away from this organism. Often, these wastes release acid, which further corrodes the intestinal-digestive lining and leads to ulcer formation.

To wash away the pain of ulcers, your goal should be to wash away the acid-releasing waste accumulation. This sludge causes what is known as "internal spontaneous combustion," which gives off noxious fumes and vapors that cause this burning of the thin membrane covering the vital digestive organs. Get rid of the sludge and you get rid of the problem of ulcers.

Cabbage Juice—Cools Acid, Promotes Healing An enzymatic substance found in freshly made cabbage juice is able to create an antacid, cooling and healing reaction often within a day or so. You need to have *fresh* cabbage. This appears to be very potent in the anti-ulcer factor. If wilted or spoiled cabbage is used, the effect is weaker. Also, you should drink the cabbage juice immediately after its preparation. Even if refrigerated for a day or so, the juice still loses its original potency. *Cooked* cabbage, although healthful, seems to lose this factor that tends to scrub away debris, cool the acid, and promote healing.

Magic Drink Ends Ulcer Distress

A gnawing ulcer pain made Morton G. a social and business loser. He rarely participated in local activities because the recurring burn in his stomach made him want to curl up in pain in the privacy of his bedroom. He became so pain-wracked, he could not devote full attention to his sales work and, understandably, it suffered. Morton G. went the route of various medications which eased the pain, but once the drug wore off, the agony returned with vengeful intensity. At times, he felt he was being "burned alive" by the churning pain. A company internist suggested he follow a simple program that helped heal and banish ulcer agony for many others—*no* seasonings of any kind in foods. Morton G. was then told to drink as many as four to six glasses of freshly prepared cabbage juice that he could make at home with an extractor. Doubtfully, he began a "no seasoning" program. Then he started to drink the juice. Immediately, he felt a soothing, balm-like contentment. Within three days, he could say goodbye and good riddance to the plague of ulcer pain. He now could enjoy a social and business round of activities. He felt as active as a teenager, thanks to the cabbage juice healing of his ulcer distress. When asked about his secret, he patted his now-soothed stomach smilingly and said it was a "magic drink." It had, indeed, performed a magic healing.

How to Chew Your Way to Ulcer Cleanliness   Thorough chewing is a unique way of causing the toxic wastes to be cleansed away. The healing of ulcers is the ultimate benefit.

Chewing releases a unique cleanser. When you chew foods, your salivary glands release an enzyme-like cleanser called *urogastrone*. This enzyme cleanser has the ability to scrub away wastes and then offer a protective balm on your intestinal lining to guard against erosion of the membrane. Chewing will also protect against volatile gastric acidity, which irritates the sore on the membrane. Therefore, you clean away the sludge and simultaneously cause healing when you use the urogastrone method. How? Simple— just chew all food thoroughly before swallowing. You'll soon be rewarded with a cleansed digestive system and a contented-cooled-cured ulcer.

Are You an Ulcer Personality?   Emotional stress (anxiety, aggravation, worry) can trigger the vagus nerve, which connects the brain with the stomach, to stimulate the secretion of excessive acid. Also, such stress causes constriction, which slows down eliminative processes and allows the buildup of harmful toxic wastes. These, too, give off acid vapors that cause erosion of the stomach lining. But not everyone who develops an ulcer is under stressful circumstances. A physiological cause, such as toxic waste accumulation, is usually the factor that gives rise to this ailment. But check your emotional condition, nevertheless. If stressful, ease up. It will help prevent a tendency toward ulcer irritation.

Ulcer-Cleansing Guidelines   Avoid these sludge-causing items: alcohol, tobacco, caffeine (coffee, tea, cola, chocolate), tea, aspirin, sugar, salt, harsh spices of any sort. These items deposit excessive amounts of waste residue that give off volatile vapors which erode the thin membrane of your stomach. You could plan to take in six small-sized meals a day instead of three full-sized ones which deposit too much toxic waste at one time for your metabolism to handle efficiently. Always begin your meal with a raw vegetable salad. End with a raw fruit. You will enable catalytic washing of your wastes to occur, thus cleansing and healing your ulcerous wounds.

Clean your digestive system and be rewarded with a sparkling metabolism that will make you glow with the joy of total youth.

SUMMARY

1. "Gluelike" accumulations in your digestive organs contribute to discomforting constipation. Wash out the glue and enjoy regularity.

2. Use a simple 25¢ fruit that will open up tight intestinal organs and promote speedy regularity.

3. Dorothy P. conquered years of toxic waste overload constipation in just three days with a simple fruit program.

4. Scrub away digestive grime with a "Miracle Salad." It gave Norah V. the look of "total youth" within four days.

5. Wash away waste-irritating indigestion on a simple six-step plan.

6. Wash away ulcers with a simple vegetable juice. Morton G. called it his "magic drink" because it ended his painful distress.

7. Chew properly and you can clean your colon while healing your ulcer through a unique enzyme reaction. Follow the basic guidelines for digestive contentment and ulcer cleansing.

CHAPTER **6**

Foods That Wash Away Overweight

Wash the fatty wastes out of your cells, and you can become slim forever. These accumulations are the root cause of your stubbornly clinging excess weight. You can break down these weight-causing toxic wastes with the use of everyday foods. These foods are able to release what is known as a catalytic enzyme reaction that helps melt and wash away the cellular wastes. This reaction is made possible when fresh raw fruits and vegetables become metabolized and begin to release fat-melting enzymes that actually scrub and scour your cells, slimming them down. So, in effect, you can *use* foods to wash away your overweight. Let's see how this reward can come about.

CELLULAR OVERLOAD—REAL CAUSE OF OVERWEIGHT

Overweight occurs when you have an excessive overload of fatty wastes that are stored primarily in your adipose (fat) cells and in your adipose (fat) tissue. These adipocytes (fatty cells and tissues) are different from ordinary cells. Most of your normal cells contain a large amount of cytoplasm (gelatin-like substance) with the cell nucleus near the center.

Fat Cells Are Different In your adipocytes or fat cells, the contents are different. Fatty wastes make up almost the entire area of the cell, and the cytoplasm and nucleus are displaced. That is, the stored-up sediment and sludge actually push out the movable cytoplasm and glue themselves to the adipocytes. More and more sludge fetters onto the already adhering sediment and weight starts to accumulate.

Obesity Continues to Expand A swelling or proliferation of adipocytes may follow, thereby increasing the amount of adipose tissue and ultimately culminating in ever-expanding obesity. To control this obesity and to help turn the tide, you need to wash away these wastes from your adipocytes. You need to slim down your cells, and your body will correspondingly slim down, too. This is the root cause of your obesity. The correction of this cause, namely fat-filled cells, will give you lifetime slimness.

FOOD ENZYMES WASH AWAY FATTY WASTES

Fresh raw fruits and vegetables and their fresh juices are highly concentrated sources of enzymes. These are the dynamic catalytic substances that have the power to break down the fatty wastes stubbornly clinging to your fat cells and help wash them out of your system. Food enzymes help scrub your fat cells and slim them down, thus slimming you down, too.

Enzymes Digest Fat-Calories-Carbohydrates When you eat or drink foods and beverages that contain high levels of fats, calories, and carbohydrates, your enzymatic system is called upon to digest these elements. If you have an abundance of enzymes, these weighty elements are metabolized and eventually eliminated. *Problem:* You may have an inadequate amount of such enzymes. This allows portions of fat, calories, and carbohydrates, in their partially metabolized forms as wastes, to be stored in your adipocytes and create excess weight.

Quick Ways to Boost Cell-Slimming Enzyme Release Your goal is to use enzymes to attack the stored-up sludge in your adipose tissue mass. You can do this by releasing more enzymes through simple eating methods. In so doing, you send forth a high concentration of these cleansers to help break down and wash out the fatty wastes clinging to your tissues. Follow these easy programs that help promote this fat-washing reaction immediately.

1. *Chew food thoroughly.* In so doing, you release salivary and digestive enzymes that can start metabolizing food even before it is swallowed. The chewing enzymes will help break down wastes and prepare them for elimination more rapidly. Salivary ptyalin digests carbohydrates and is activated with thorough chewing.

2. *Be cautious about refined sweeteners.* Sugar in any form creates a neutralization of valuable enzymes and renders them either weak or helpless. Refined sugar will be absorbed speedily by your body with hardly any digestive action. The waste residues then cling to your adipocytes and cause billowing overweight in no time at all. Avoid refined sweeteners.

3. *Do not drown enzymes with liquids at mealtime.* Your enzymes function more vigorously in cell cleansing if they are not drenched with liquid consumed before, during, or after mealtime. You run the risk of *diluting* these enzymes and reducing their cell-cleansing power. Therefore, plan to drink any liquid two hours *before* your meal. Do not drink with meals. Drink two hours *after* your meal. This gives full power to your enzymes in cell cleansing.

4. *Avoid temperature extremes in foods and beverages.* Too hot or too cold foods and beverages can either scald or freeze your digestive enzymes. Such temperature extremes can also deactivate vital digestive processes so that cellular overload increases. Make sure that whatever you consume is at a comfortable taste temperature. This makes it soothing for your enzymatic process.

5. *Avoid sharp seasonings.* Salt, pepper, monosodium glutamate, and related volatile seasonings "burn" enzymes and practically destroy them. These sharp flavorings leave waste residue behind which then becomes glued to your adipocytes. Worse, they are sponge-like and suck up liquids, thereby becoming bloated. You gain excessive weight because of this liquid-engorged salt residue. Use more flavorful (and mild) herbs for cleaner taste and cleaner cells, too.

23 FOODS THAT WASH AWAY YOUR OVERWEIGHT

Here is a list of 23 high-enzyme foods that get to the root cause of your overweight, namely, washing away the accumulated wastes from your adipocytes. When you eat these foods, your thorough chewing releases enzymes that work speedily to break down the stubborn wastes that are glued to your adipocytes. You can actually eat your way to a lifetime slimness with these cell-cleansing foods.

Suggested Program: Eat several of these foods daily, preferably raw. If cooking is required, steam just long enough until they are tender for chewing. Eat them in combination or singly. If seasoning is desired, use a little lemon juice, a sprinkle of apple cider vinegar, or desired herbs.

For powerful super-cell cleansing action, plan to *begin* each meal with several of these cell-washing enzyme vegetables. In this way, they will be available for digesting the fat, calories, and carbohydrates from the foods that follow. These enzyme vegetables help control the amount of waste that will then be deposited on your adipocytes. In effect, you can eat your way to slimness on this simple program.

Remember to chew all foods thoroughly.

Asparagus	Collards	Parsley
Beans (green)	Cucumber	Romaine Lettuce
Broccoli	Dandelion Greens	Squash
Brussels Sprouts	Escarole	Swiss Chard
Carrots	Kale	Tomato
Cauliflower	Lettuce	Turnip Greens
Celery	Mushrooms	Watercress
Chicory	Mustard Greens	

Sheds 34 Pounds, Shrinks 9 Inches, Within 14 Weeks

Unpleasingly plump Beth Z. waddled instead of walked, spread instead of sat, billowed in whatever she wore. She had a lifetime problem with excess weight. And even worse, it kept increasing. She desperately sought help from a bariatrician (physician who specializes in obesity) who suggested she get to the cause of her problem, namely, the weighty wastes that clung to her adipocytes. He put her on a simple enzyme program. Beth Z. was told to begin each meal with a variety of the listed 23 high-enzyme foods. This would set off an immediate enzymatic action that would (1) wash her fat-filled cells and (2) metabolize and fully digest eaten foods. This would protect against waste deposition in her cells. She was also told to control caloric intake and eliminate refined sugar in any form. Results? The pounds just melted away. Beth Z. saw the scales go down, down, down. Amazed, she was able to shed 34 stubborn pounds, shrink 9 unsightly inches, and all within 14 weeks. She soon became a lovely 120-pound woman with a neat figure. She was able to be *permanently* slim with the simple practice of eating a raw salad before each meal for enzyme slimming.

Simple Six-Step Raw Food Plan   The million-dollar health spas of exclusive resorts worldwide charge top dollar to overweight clients from the top echelons of society to follow this simple program. You can do it right at home. It consists of a six-step plan that you follow on *alternate* days of the week. In between, follow the enzyme-enhancing programs outlined in this chapter and throughout the book. You will notice that fat is washing right out of your cells as the scales drop and your inches melt. Here is this million-dollar cell-washing plan.

1. *Morning Meal.* Have a plate of fresh fruit in season for breakfast. Select any desired fruit in any favorite combinations. You must chew carefully before you swallow. Eat leisurely. Fruit should not be ice cold but a comfortable cool temperature.

2. *Mid-Morning Snack.* Drink one or two glasses of either fresh fruit or vegetable juice.

3. *Noon Meal.* Eat a plate of fresh raw vegetables in season. Select any desired combination. Eat leisurely and chew thoroughly. Vegetables should not be ice cold, either; keep them at an enzyme-soothing cool temperature.

4. *Mid-Afternoon Snack.* Drink one or two glasses of either fresh fruit or vegetable juice.

5. *Evening Meal.* Make a platter of different raw vegetables than those enjoyed earlier, and chew thoroughly.

6. *Late-Evening Snack.* Drink a glass of fresh vegetable juice. Its high natural mineral content is soothing and helps you sleep soundly.

Works While You Sleep   Throughout the day, you have spared your fat-melting digestive system the responsibility of heavier, cooked foods. Without this interference, enzymes now focus full force on your adipose (fat) cells, and dislodging the weighty wastes that are responsible for your obesity. Within an hour after you finish the meal or snack, a treasure of waste-washing enzymes are breaking up cell sludge vigorously and starting the slimming process. This continues throughout the night, while you sleep, since the powerful enzymes do not have to share responsibilities with heavier and cooked foods.

The next morning, you can see and feel the weight loss via your scales and mirror. The pounds and inches are shrinking because the catalytic enzymes have loosened and dissolved the fat from your adipose tissues.

Alternate Days for Raw Food Fast   The million-dollar spas prescribe this dynamic cell-shrinking raw food fast for alternate days. On the in-between days, eat healthfully and with common sense. When your weight has reached a desired level, you may limit the raw food fast program to one day a week. The spa specialists suggest a "maintenance" program of one fast every ten days. It keeps your catalytic enzymes in tiptop shape as they keep your cells in slim shape, too.

From "Fat" to "Slim" in One Weekend

When Jeff X.'s insurance company wanted to cancel his policy because of his increasing corpulence, he had to act swiftly. The company physician, who had studied the miraculous weight-losing programs of health spas, told Jeff X. to follow a three-day weekend raw food program. Anxious to shed his undesirable weight, Jeff X. tried the regimen. It was pleasing because he liked to "chew on something" while dieting. Other diets left him unsatisfied, but chewing raw fruits and vegetables did give him the pleasure he rightfully deserved. Almost at once, his adipose cells started to shrink. Within two days, the pounds and inches started coming off. When he finished the weekend, he had shed so much unwanted weight, he was dubbed "Slim" (he used to be called "Fat" behind his back) and was accepted for insurance renewal. It took just one weekend for this miracle to happen.

TWO SIMPLE STEPS THAT PROTECT AGAINST CELLULAR OVERWEIGHT

Why Are Cells Overloaded?   Briefly, when you consume calories from fats, proteins, and carbohydrates, these substances are transformed into *adenosine triphosphate* or ATP. This waste product is then deposited in your cells if not properly burned off at the time of intake. Therefore, your cells become overweight because of the stored-up ATP.

How to Reduce Cells? Provide enzymatic energy that will enter the cells and dislodge the ATP waste, and thereby start cellular slimming. Enzymes are the devices needed to bring about this melting away of the ATP wastes from your cells.

To provide cell-slimming enzymes that "attack" the stubborn ATP clumps, follow these two simple steps:

1. Begin each meal with a raw vegetable platter. *Benefit:* Carefully chewed vegetables provide both digestive and food enzymes, which actually "shower" the cells and wash away the ATP clumps.

2. Finish each meal with a raw fruit platter. *Benefit:* Ingested foods, with their high caloric waste deposition, will not be allowed to remain when fruit enzymes drive forth to uproot and wash them out of the system right after the meal.

Easy, Effective, Enzymatic This easy change is effective quickly with the enzymatic dispatchers that work right on the spot to nip cellular overweight right in the bud.

Eats and Loses Weight with Two-Step Plan

Years of cellular overloading had made Judy O'H. "hopelessly" fat. Then a nutrition counselor suggested she follow the simple two-step plan to boost release of ATP cell-slimming enzymes. Judy O'H. did cut down on portions and fats, but she still ate wholesomely with just these simple changes: a raw vegetable platter before a meal to send forth enzymes, and a raw fruit platter after a meal to double enzymatic catalytic action upon ingested food. Result? She could eat and still shrink down her weight almost at once. Over 40 pounds "disappeared" this way. And the joy of it was that Judy O'H. could still eat most of her favorite foods . . . as long as she used the vegetable-fruit program. It was the most delicious diet she ever followed, and it worked!

SAY "NO" TO THESE WASTE-CAUSING FOODS

Put the red "stop" light on these danger foods. They add cement-like sludge to your adipose cells and harden to such a thickness, it would require Herculean enzymes to get them off. Avoid this problem by avoiding these waste-causing foods: soft drinks, chocolate, candy, jellies, jams, ice cream, soda, sundaes, doughnuts, cookies, cakes, pies, sugar, pretzels, potato chips, gravies, fried foods, sugar-coated cereals, sweetened fruit drinks and ades and colas, bacon, fatty meats, sausages, alcoholic drinks, salt.

In Brief: Whatever contains either "sugar" or "salt" is a "no-no." These are dangerous sources of thick sludge on your cells. Avoid such waste-causing foods and you will avoid cellular overload and body overweight.

You can wash the weight right out of your cells by eating the right foods and beverages and avoiding the wrong ones. You'll discover that you can actually eat your way to a slim-trim figure and a more youthful body, too.

HIGHLIGHTS

1. Cellular overload, the real root cause of overweight, can be conquered with the intake of raw food enzymes.
2. Boost cell-slimming enzyme release with the basic five-step plan.
3. Eat freely of the 23 foods that actually wash away your overweight.
4. Beth Z. shed 34 pounds, shrank 9 inches within 14 weeks by eating of these 23 foods, in any desired combination or quantity.
5. The million-dollar health spas offer a six-step raw food plan that works miracles in creating dramatic weight loss.
6. Jeff X. went from "fat" to "slim" in one weekend on an easy raw food plan.
7. Two simple steps used by Judy O'H. gave her dramatic weight loss.

CHAPTER 7

Say Goodbye to Allergies with Cellular Washing

With each breath you take, you deposit an overwhelming amount of toxic pollutants on the millions of cells and tissues that make up your respiratory organs. These waste particles need to be washed away constantly so that your oxygen exchange will be free of blockage. But in a polluted environment, as well as with the intake of chemically treated foods, toxic wastes tend to overwhelm the usual self-cleansing process and respiratory pollution starts to take hold.

ALLERGY-CAUSING INTERNAL POLLUTION

As toxic wastes accumulate, they swell up the lining membranes of your bronchial tubes. Internal pollution causes contraction of the surrounding musculature and plugs up the tubes by depositing more and more waste particles. Thick mucus is another form of lung pollution. If these wastes are allowed to accumulate, they may predispose toward conditions of asthma, serious coughs, extreme dust sensitivities, seasonal allergies (hay fever, for example), and annoying shortness of breath. This last-named problem can cause such an oxygen deficiency that cardiovascular distress may eventually occur. So you can see that toxic wastes allowed to stick to your bronchial tubes can shorten your very breath of life!

Check Your Own Breathing Problem Are there times when you appear to be gasping for air? Even if you climb a small staircase, does it leave you breathless? You may have trouble *exhaling,* more so than *inhaling.* What's the difference? Exhalation difficulties tell you that the air passages of your small bronchii have become clogged with waste particles and constricted with toxic-like mucus, thus squeezing the passages. This makes it hard for you to breathe *out.* It is a sign that your breathing apparatus has become overloaded with toxic wastes and you need to use methods of cellular washing so that you can say goodbye to the choking, sputtering, desperate need for precious air. These all-natural methods can be followed right in the privacy of your own home. They work swiftly and effectively to help you get rid of allergy-causing wastes.

ONE-DAY JUICE FAST = FREEDOM FROM ALLERGIES

The accumulated glue-like sludge that has fastened to your bronchial tubes needs to be jarred loose and prepared for elimination so you can free yourself from this irritation. This can be done through the powerful detoxifying powers of *lemon juice.*

The high concentration of bioflavonoids as well as enzymes and Vitamin C, together with natural fruit acids, have the power to dislodge, break down and disintegrate toxic wastes that have glued themselves to your lungs.

How to Prepare: In a glass of freshly boiled water, squeeze the juice of one or two fresh lemons. Add a dab of honey, if desired. Stir slowly. When tepid, drink this cleansing lemonade.

How Much to Drink: Throughout the day, take no other foods or beverages (except water, but keep to a minimum). Instead, drink up to six or even eight glasses of this lemon juice cleanser. This is an effective lung-washing juice fast.

Cleanses Lungs, Washes Cells   The vigorous enzymes will break down accumulated wastes, and then use the natural Vitamin C content to help rebuild the collagen and cellular walls so that they are strong enough to resist the onslaught of continuous pollution. Your lungs become cleansed; your cells are washed and restored. Sparkling clean, they now enable you to breathe more healthfully.

Simple Program: Depending upon the severity of your lung pollution, you should plan on having a one-day lemon juice fast every seven days. As your bronchial tubes become cleansed, as the debris is scrubbed away and your breathing is easier, you may reduce the frequency of the lemon juice fast. Thereafter, schedule this cell-washing fast twice a month for lifetime freedom from allergic upset.

Conquers Hopeless Asthma in Two Days with Juice Fast

A victim of childhood asthma, Alma DeB. was told that her case was "hopeless" and that she would have to live with her breathing problem. She chose, instead, to try to find a way to live without this choking affliction. A naturopathic physician said that an examination showed her bronchial tubes to be covered with long-accumulated glue-like wastes. They had so irritated her fragile respiratory cells, that any particle inhaled would bring about an asthmatic attack.

Alma DeB. was told to go on a two-day lemon juice fast. She was allowed no other foods or beverages but up to eight glasses of this warm lemon juice drink. *Reason:* the lemon substances would work without interference from other ingested foods or liquids. Almost at once, Alma DeB. was able to breathe easier. By the middle of the second day, the lemon juice had so cleansed her bronchial tubes, she could breathe deeply with welcome comfort. By the end of the second day, she had fully recovered. Thereafter, she never again had an asthma attack. To be on the safe side, she cleans her bronchial cells and tissues with a lemon juice fasting program just once every ten days. It helps her say "goodbye forever" to her asthma allergy attacks.

CLEAN UP YOUR LIFESTYLE AND CLEAN UP YOUR BREATHING ORGANS

Constant Waste Dumping   Air pollution, cigarette smoke (not necessarily your own), crowded living and working conditions all deposit wastes upon your breathing organs. You inhale close to 3,000 gallons of air per day. This air can cause a constant waste dumping on your lungs. These toxic pollutants include carbon dioxide, carbon monoxide, hydrogen sulfide, hydrocarbons from auto exhausts, asbestos, carbon particulates, rubber compounds. The list is endless. These pollutants actually "choke" your breathing organs with the constant dumping of wastes.

Little Chance of Escape   Rural areas have less pollutants but still are not as safe as you would wish them to be. Winds carry wastes from industrial and crowded areas for hundreds of miles from the original source. Country living offers little escape from the constant intake of waste-accumulating pollutants.

Build Resistance at Home   The answer here is to build within yourself as much resistance to lung pollution as possible. You can begin right at home. By cleaning your lifestyle, you will help clean up your breathing organs. You can enjoy more than allergy freedom; you can hope for a healthier and longer lifetime. Start now to bring about these changes at home.

1. Remove everything that gives off unpleasant odors. Keep them out of inhalation range until absolutely required for use and then use only in a ventilated area. Pollution-causing items include furniture polishes, window and oven cleaners, insecticides, cosmetics, hair sprays, nail polish and remover, paint in any form, commercial glues, medications, etc. All give off fumes that seep through containers and right into your lungs. Out of scent . . . out of your lungs.

2. Have your automatic stove pilot light turned off, professionally, if need be. It is a constant source of indoor pollution and gas seepage. Keep gas use to an absolute minimum, whether at the stove or dryer or heater.

3. Check food wrappings carefully. *Caution:* plastic containers (whether cardboard-like or flexible) are heat-sealed onto the food. Pollutants leak forth and contaminate the food. Wherever possible, opt for fresh foods as much as you can. Glass enclosed products are good, too.

4. If you want to keep clean and look good then use more natural products. Use ordinary baking soda (with or without a pinch of salt) as a dentrifice and mouth wash. Men, try an electric razor. For an astringent, use ordinary ice water. Use baby soaps and baby shampoos because they're much milder and less polluting than the adult variety. Replace any plastic containers with glass—even cardboard is preferable.

5. Clothing should be washed in a detergent-free biodegradable washing soda or soap. Otherwise, the chemicals in washing materials and rinses, etc., cling to the garments and then penetrate into your pores. *Simple Test:* Sprinkle a few drops of water on a

ready-to-wear garment. If the water penetrates through, the garment is healthy to wear. If it remains on top, the garment is chemically polluted and you would do well to avoid its use. Tip: Read garment labels. Select items that are pure natural cloth (cotton, wool, etc.) without any synthetics.

6. Restrict or eliminate any use of rubber. That includes plastic foam. Bedding should be as natural as possible. Sheets, pillow cases, blankets should all be of a natural material. Avoid the use of polyester for bedding since the warmth of your body will release its hydrocarbons which then enter your open pores to create internal pollution. *Caution:* Avoid use of an electric blanket. Yes, it is warm, but its wires are sealed in plastic and when heated will give off an invisible vapor that enters your body. Instead, garb yourself in woolen nightclothes.

7. Cookwear should be stainless steel, cast iron, copper, but *not* aluminum. Heating aluminum gives off noxious waste-laden fumes. Avoid frying because it causes formation of tars on foods and also indoor pollution.

8. Wash pots and dishes with tap water and any soap that is detergent-free or biodegradable. Use the same type of washing soda. Rinse thoroughly. *Caution:* Do not use paper towels because they are coated with chemicals and various chlorine bleaches. Remember to *avoid* plastics of any sort, and that includes cookwear and serving wear, too.

9. Check all of your heating systems and exhaust fans. In just one hour (at 350°F.) your gas oven can give off concentrations of carbon monoxide and nitrogen dioxide that can actually cause an allergic attack. Make certain your exhaust fans work perfectly. Always keep windows open to let fumes escape.

10. Keep your living and working quarters clean and dry. Avoid dampness because it is a breeding site for molds and spores that can be inhaled and coat your lungs until you develop allergic attacks.

Remember, such toxic wastes can penetrate your mucous secretions, be swallowed, and then be taken up via your intestinal tract, leading to rising levels of body pollution. Make these basic adjustments in your lifestyle and you will be able to breathe better in a life-giving style.

ALTERNATE NOSTRIL BREATHING TECHNIQUE
FOR INTERNAL CLEANSING

Your Nose: Body's Air-Conditioner   The mucous membranes of your nasal cavities have the ability to promote body air-conditioning. Inhalation programs can cause a freer exchange of air so that there is a more vigorous dislodging and subsequent removal of accumulated pollutants.

The suction that is used during a unique method known as "alternate nostril breathing" will help draw pollutants out of your respiratory tract and thereby promote an important cleansing reaction. This can be done easily at home or wherever you have just five minutes to yourself. It helps decongest your respiratory organs and enables you to breathe easier.

Asthma, Sensitivities, Coughs Are Relieved   This "alternate nostril breathing" program is able to discharge enough irritants so that there is speedy relief from asthmatic attacks, sensitivities to dust, and stubborn coughs. To boost results, plan to use this method (1) whenever you feel a breathing problem threatening to take hold, and (2) as a maintenance program, at least once or twice each day.

Four-Step Program

1. Breathe in through both sides of your nose. Breathe out through one side, closing your other nostril with your finger.
2. Breathe in and out through the same side, closing the other side with your finger.
3. Breathe in through the side that is less blocked. Breathe out through the other side, closing the unused nostril with your finger.
4. If both sides are blocked? Breathe in through your mouth and out through one side of your nose as forcibly as necessary. As soon as one side of your nose opens sufficiently to allow it, then breathe in through the open side. Stop the mouth breathing.

Suggestion: Just five minutes of this "alternate nostril breathing" method each day will help control the inner pollutant level and more important, help wash out those irritating wastes. You'll find it easier and more refreshing to breathe better. You will also find yourself building greater immunity to allergic distress. In due time, allergies will be washed away!

Breathes Free and Overcomes Allergies in Five Days

Construction engineer Morton Y.S. would suffer from choked breath when climbing just a few steps. On the job site, he turned blue, gasped for air, and sputtered with his tongue hanging out after walking just a short distance. His condition so worsened that just a slight bit of dust or pollution gave him a stuffed nose in minutes. This almost asphyxiated him. Such a disability threatened his job. The company respiratory specialists suggested that he help wash away the breath-choking pollution with the "alternate nostril breathing" method. Morton Y.S. took frequent "breathing breaks" as he called them. About four times daily, he would use the method. Within five days, he could breathe freely. He overcame his allergies. Now, he can work (and breathe) with the vigor of a youngster!

WHISTLE YOUR WAY TO CLEANER LUNGS

Just as your normal breathing power sucks in pollution and deposits stubborn grime upon your lungs, so can the reverse method help remove these allergy-causing wastes. You can do this with a very easy trick—*whistling.*

25¢ Whistle = Million Dollar Throat   At any toy store, get yourself a whistle. It costs about 25¢ or even less. Whenever you are out of earshot, just whistle! The forceful blowing will create a vacuum cleaner effect on your lungs. Dirt will be uprooted and cast out. *Suggestion:* To silence the whistle, remove the little pit-like nuggets.

Using a whistle (whether silent or chirping) causes you to *pucker* your lips. This improves the vacuum effect and is more vigorous in uprooting and casting out cell-eroding wastes. Whistle as often as possible for speedy lung cleansing.

The breath of life should do exactly that—give you life. Protect your body against cellular congestion and the choking agony of allergic attacks with these cleansing programs. Breathing will then provide refreshing nourishment and youthful vigor. You will then be able to say goodbye forever to so-called "hopeless" allergies.

MAIN POINTS

1. Nip lung congestion in the bud with a one-day lemon juice fast. It washes away accumulated debris and helps you breathe better.
2. Alma DeB. conquered hopeless asthma in two days with this juice fast.
3. Clean up your lifestyle with tips offered for cleaner breathing organs.
4. Air-condition your body with "alternate nostril breathing" techniques.
5. Morton Y.S. overcame allergies in five days with a breathing method.
6. Whistling (quietly, please) is a simple and fun way to clean your lungs and protect against allergies.

8

How to Supercharge Your Heart with Youthful Power . . . While You Sleep!

Cleanse your heart while you sleep and you will experience a feeling of renewed vitality upon awakening. With the use of proper foods and programs that you perform during the day, the internal cleansing process will be able to wash away debris from your heart and arteries throughout the night. A catalytic reaction begins that metabolizes and removes wastes through the natural eliminative channels. When you wake up, you will have a clean heart and a longer lifeline, too.

HOW TOXEMIA CAN CONTRIBUTE TO HEART DISTRESS

To understand how internal washing can benefit your heart while you sleep, it is helpful to know just how toxemia is a threat to cardiac (and total body) health. This will make it much easier for you to use the programs involved in "heart washing."

Sneaky Sludge Threatens Heart Health Accumulated wastes are "sneaky" because they tend to cling together and form heart-threatening sludge over a period of time, without your awareness. These wastes, from the wrong foods and from environmental pollution, cling to the arteries of your body. Gradually, the inner walls of the arteries become thickened and irregular with more and more deposits of these fatty waste substances. Called *atheromata*, these fatty wastes accumulate slowly in your blood vessels. If they are not washed out, they block the blood vessel and this causes cardiovascular trouble. It may cause an occlusion (waste blockage) or a more serious arteriosclerosis of the cerebral vessels.

Therefore, the key to protection against these disabling penalties for allowing sludge to accumulate is to embark upon a simple but effective cleansing program as early as possible.

INTERNAL WASHING PROTECTS AGAINST HEART ATTACK

By keeping your heart cleansed, you can protect it against the threat of an attack. How is this possible? The answer is that when your two most important blood vessels (right and left coronary arteries which begin at the base of the aorta, or large artery that carries blood from your heart to all body parts) become blocked with fatty waste deposits.

This blockage denies the heart muscle its needed oxygen and nutrients. So the heart muscle actually dies! This is the start of the sludge-causing problem. The dead heart muscle is surrounded by an area of acute injury and an area of temporary injury or waste-causing inflammation called an *infarction*. This injured area causes the heart to lose some of its effectiveness as a pump because there is less muscle to contract and force blood out.

Sludge Pile-Up Worsens Problem   As more and more wastes are allowed to pile up, they increase blood pressure and contribute to an irregular heart rate. The sludge reduces your body's oxygen-carrying abilities, thus denying your heart the needed supply of oxygen. The buildup of carbon monoxide in the blood also boosts the risk of clots that could block the heart. As sludge mounts up, the heart becomes so choked, it is vulnerable to a heart attack.

"WASTE-FORMING" VS. "WASTE-CLEANING" FOODS

There are two basic groupings of foods; one group can lead to waste formation, and the other group to waste cleaning. Plan your eating program to cut down on the waste-forming foods and boost intake of waste-cleaning foods. Here is a simple guideline to help you be good to your heart.

Limit intake of foods that are "waste-forming" for your heart, such as: dairy foods that contain fat, fatty meats such as beef, pork, lamb, regular hamburger, ground chuck, fatty and very-marbled cuts of meat, oil-packed foods (mayonnaise or salad dressing), butter, hydrogenated products, egg yolks (eaten without whites), sugar, salt and products made with these flavorings, chemically treated foods.

Increase intake of "waste-cleaning" foods for your heart. These include: fresh fruits and vegetables in any variety and quantity, their fresh juices, seeds, nuts, foods made with whole grains, very lean animal foods, egg whites, fat-free dairy products.

Watch for "Hidden" Fatty Wastes   This includes the butter or margarine on your bread and vegetables, the oil used to fry your favorite foods, the chunks of white fat on your meat that you want to trim off, but too often eat. But that's not all; many foods contain fatty wastes that you cannot see; whole milk, hard cheese, ice cream, and "marbled" meats contain such wastes. Restrict or eliminate intake of these fatty waste foods and you will help control sludge that threatens to choke the life out of your heart.

CLEANSE YOUR HEART WHILE YOU SLEEP

During the day, for your scheduled meals, plan to take in large quantities of fresh fruits and vegetables, moderate amounts of whole grains, legumes, a small portion of a skim milk product, and several glasses of fresh fruit and vegetable juices.

Catalytic Reaction Works Overnight   The high concentration of catalytic enzymes in the raw foods will become stimulated by the invigorating vitamins and minerals in the others. They will dislodge and break down the accumulated deposits that otherwise cling stubbornly to the inner walls of your arteries. The enzymes will initiate a thermal cauterization reaction wherein they actually melt away the porridge-like toxic waste accumulation and help prepare it for elimination. This works while you sleep!

From "Choked Breath" to "Vitality" Within 48 Hours

Henry O'H. was a sedentary bookkeeper and this inactivity may have contributed to his toxic waste overload. He would consume large amounts of the "waste-forming" foods which deposited excessive amounts of sludge on his cardiovascular system so that he had "choked breath" reactions and a pale skin. At times, his heart pounded so furiously, he thought it would burst. An exam by his cardiologist revealed this dangerous accumulation. A program was suggested for quick relief. Henry also felt sluggish and overburdened because of this restriction of free oxygen nourishment to his heart, so he was told to devote three days a week to the "waste-cleaning" foods. The remaining four days included his usual diet, but fats, salt, sugar, artificial flavorings were taboo. Henry O'H. immediately followed this easy cleansing program. Results: overnight, the deposits became loosened and were ready for elimination by morning. Within 48 hours, he could breathe healthfully. He had rejuvenated vitality, too. He realized that a clean heart had given him a clean body and a more youthful source of energy.

GARLIC: AMAZING TOTAL HEART CLEANSER

This potent vegetable has an amazing reaction, which uproots and then casts out the fatty wastes that threaten the health of your heart and your entire body.

Secret of Heart-Cleansing Power   Garlic contains a rich concentration of allicin. This is an active sulfur-containing substance that is transformed by your metabolism into a unique sludge-washing substance called diallyldisulfide. Your enzymatic system uses this substance to chip away, break down, melt, and actually dissolve the porridge-like wastes that stubbornly cling to your cardiovascular system. This is the astonishing secret of garlic's heart-cleansing power.

Controls Cholesterol, Dilutes Thick Fats   This same garlic activator, diallyldisulfide, has the ability to cleanse deposits from your bloodstream and thereby lower your serum cholesterol levels. This garlic "scrubber" is able to synthesize or break down wastes and fatty deposits in your liver. Therefore, there is an overall reduction of wastes in your bloodstream and your heart. Garlic also brings about a reduction in the deposition levels of triglycerides (other forms of fatty wastes) in your bloodstream and this protects you from toxic overload that could predispose heart trouble. Garlic is the flavorful protector of your heart . . . and life.

How to Use Heart-Washing Garlic   Either chew several cloves daily, or chop a garlic bulb very finely and add to a salad, stew, casserole, soup, or main dish. You may also press out garlic juice (a special garlic press is available at many health stores and housewares outlets) and mix with a glass of vegetable juice. Drink one glass daily. The garlic compounds work vigorously and speedily to bring down your toxic levels and protect your heart from corrosive attack.

Garlic at Night = Heart Health at Daybreak   About two hours before going to sleep, consume four or five cloves of garlic. (Remember to chew parsley to neutralize the pungent odor.) Or else, chop finely and add to a raw lettuce and tomato salad. Eat this before retiring for the night.

While You Sleep: The active elements in the garlic work with a super-energy because your basic processes are now at rest. Therefore, undiluted energy can be mustered for the heart-scrubbing reaction. During your eight hours of sleep, the garlic compounds are washing away toxic wastes. Upon awakening, you'll have a cleaner heart and a more youthful vitality, too.

THE SUPER-CLEANSING FOOD THAT DOUBLES YOUR HEART POWER

A small amount of an amazingly powerful super-cleansing food is able to dilute and discharge the most obstructive sludge deposits from your cardiovascular system and give your heart twice as much youthful power. It works immediately.

Meet This Super-Cleanser   The name is *lecithin* (pronounced less-i-thin); it is a bland, water-soluble granular powder made from de-fatted soybeans. Cardiologists call it a *phosphatide,* which is a vital waste-cleansing substance that should be available to all living cells, tissues, organs.

Lecithin's secret is in its *phospholipid* power. This power enables this wonder food to melt away stubborn fats and wastes and thereby cleanse your cardiovascular system.

The amazing power of lecithin is its function as an emulsifier. It keeps fats and wastes broken up into microscopic particles so that they can be removed through arterial walls. *Protective Factor:* Lecithin searches out and then breaks down the plaques (fibrous clumps that stick to your cardiovascular system) so they can be washed right out of your body. Lecithin is your super-cleansing heart food.

STIMULATE INTERNAL CLEANSING IN MINUTES

Lecithin—Your Heart Cleanser   Your heart requires a special enzyme called *lecithin cholesterol acyltransferase* (LCAT) in order to control the accumulation of waste on arterial walls. LCAT acts as a scrubber in that it keeps wastes from gluing together, and keeps them emulsified and prepared for elimination.

Special Need: In order for your body to make this self-scrubbing LCAT, it requires lecithin. With this super-food, a special cleansing action takes place. Lecithin causes body substances to act as intracellular "bouncers" that displace and discharge undesirable wastes and fatty plaques. It becomes your heart-saver . . . and life-saver, too.

Easy Way to Obtain Cleansing Lecithin   Available at health stores, choose the lecithin granules. These are of top quality. They offer you the highest potency of phosphatides and phosphatidyl choline, which are the powerhouses behind the scrubbing action. So, for top-cleansing results, use the granules.

How to Use: At breakfast, add four tablespoons of the granules to your breakfast cereal. At noontime, sprinkle two tablespoons over your fruit or vegetable salad. At dinnertime, add four tablespoons to your main dish or your salad.

Swift Reaction: Within moments after swallowing, the scrubbing substances in lecithin begin to cleanse your arteries and heart. You'll start to feel better almost at once. They continue scrubbing *overnight*. You will wake up feeling younger, thanks to lecithin.

You Can See the Scrubbing Power of Lecithin   When you roast a fatty cut of meat, let the juices collect in a pan and cool off. Note that the fatty globules rise to the top. Now sprinkle one tablespoon of lecithin on top of the fat. Wait for 20 to 30 minutes. You'll discover that the fat has *disappeared!* The juices are there, but where is the fat? The lecithin has emulsified the fat, broken down the wastes and prepared them for speedy disposal.

The same cleansing action occurs when you use lecithin in your meals. It will break up plaques and promote a scrubbing power that will give you a cleaner cardiovascular system almost overnight.

Simple Program: Plan to use eight to ten tablespoons of lecithin granules daily. Gradually, as you experience improved heart health, better oxygenation, and better energy, your intake can be lowered to four tablespoons daily. Simple and tasty, these granules offer you a heart-scrubbing and artery-cleansing reaction that just cannot be equalled. Lecithin may well be the super-food that will give you a clean heart . . . and a healthier lifestyle.

Cleans "Choked" Heart Within 48 Hours

Shortness of breath, palpitations of the heart, chest tightening all made Nora DeL. fearful that she was developing cardiac difficulties. A physiologist told this housewife that she had accumulations of waste plaques that needed to be eliminated immediately. He suggested she omit the waste-forming foods from animal sources, and boost the waste-washing foods from plant sources. But on top of it all, she was told to take just 10 tablespoons of lecithin granules throughout the day. Nora DeL. wanted swift action. She immediately took the granules, about 3 tablespoons with each meal. Some 48 hours later, she returned to the physiologist. It was amazing. The sludge had been washed right out of her body. She could breathe more deeply, enjoyed a smoothly functioning heart and a "comfortable" chest, free of fearsome pains. All this happened within 48 hours. Nora DeL. has lecithin to thank for freeing her "choked" heart and giving her a healthier life to come.

AN ONION A DAY KEEPS YOUR HEART DOCTOR AWAY

Shed no tears over the pungent onion. Instead, be grateful for this aromatic food because it has the power of cleansing your heart with such thoroughness, it can help keep your heart doctor away.

Melts Fats, Cleans, and Breaks Down Sludge   The onion contains enzymes that are able to melt away accumulated fats and scrub them right out of your cardiovascular system. These onion enzymes are also able to shrink down plaque-like fibrin which might otherwise induce a dangerous blood clot.

The onion contains a hormone-like substance known as a prostaglandin. It uses this ingredient to clean out sludge from your blood and thereby control the vigor of your heart beat.

Onion compounds reduce platelet aggregation sludge by breaking down a dangerous waste called thromboxane. By suppressing the multiplication of this waste, onion enzymes cause internal washing so that you are protected from heart distress. Onion enzymes also break up the "dams" of small blood clots called thrombi which could otherwise gather and induce a heart attack. Just eating onions daily can help your body maintain this self-cleansing heart action.

Look (If You Can) at the Waste-Washing Power of Onions   Just start to slice up a fresh onion or two. In moments, your eyes start to water. The aroma of this all-powerful cleanser is so pungent that without even touching your eyes, it stimulates your lacrimal glands to release tears that wash away debris from your sight organs. The same reaction occurs when you *eat* onions. Their enzymes cause a melting down and washing out of accumulated debris. Like internal sprinklers, the enzymes wash and cleanse your cardiovascular system and eliminate the sludge. Just eat onions for this internal heart-washing action to occur.

Onion Eating Plan   Plan to use any seasonal raw onions as part of a vegetable salad daily. Or, use onions in cooking. Their cleansing powers are evident when cooked, too. Are you bothered because they make you weep on the outside when you would prefer this weeping (cleansing) inside? Then refrigerate the onion before slicing to inhibit its tear-inducing powers. Or, cut the onion under water for the same benefit. Eat one to two onions as part of your vegetable plan each day. Your heart will be all the cleaner.

"ALL-NATURAL HEART CLEANSING TONIC"

In a tall glass of fresh vegetable juice, add two tablespoons of lecithin granules, and one sliced or diced onion. Blenderize. Drink one glass daily.

Revives Heart, Boosts Health in Three Days

Chest weakness and difficulty in breathing made Phyllis MacB. fearful that her heart was acting up on her. Since three family members had cardiac difficulties, she thought she would be next. Her internist said the problem stemmed from her clogged arterioles and heart valves. He put Phyllis MacB. on a waste-washing program of eating more plant foods. He also prescribed the "All-Natural Heart Cleansing Tonic," to be taken twice daily. Within one day, Phyllis MacB. could breathe better. Her chest weakness was overcome, and she had more youthful energy. At the end of three days, she was tested again. Her internist said she had been so cleansed, she had the heart health of a youngster. She resumed her regular activities with a new (and longer) lease on life.

How Tonic Creates Speedy Heart Cleansing The vitamin-mineral-enzyme combination of the vegetables invigorates the fat-fighting powers of the lecithin. The same vegetable combo will use the onion prostaglandin to promote accelerated heart cleansing. Within moments after swallowing, this double-cleansing action takes place. It works, often overnight, to give you a super-clean heart the next morning. And it's a refreshingly tasty tonic, too!

Heart Clogged at Nightfall, Heart Cleansed at Daybreak By following these programs, your clogged heart can be cleansed by daybreak—overnight! Just give your body the working materials required for this miracle cleansing action. Your heart will then last nine lives and then some.

SUMMARY

1. A clean heart is a healthy heart. Avoid sludge-forming foods in order to add years to your life.
2. Limit or eliminate "waste-forming" foods and boost intake of "waste-cleaning" foods. They wash your heart while you sleep!
3. Henry O'H. used the beneficial cleaning foods to go from "choked breath" to vitality within 48 hours.
4. Garlic is a dynamic heart-cleanser. Take it at night and have a healthier heart by morning.

5. Lecithin is a super-cleansing food for your heart and total body.

6. Nora DeL. was able to clean her "choked" heart within 48 hours with a dietary change and the use of lecithin.

7. The humble onion is a powerful heart-cleanser. In combination with lecithin, in an "All-Natural Heart Cleansing Tonic," it revived Phyllis MacB. within three days.

CHAPTER **9**

Miracle Power Foods
for Dynamic Circulation

If you wash away toxic accumulations you will wake up your sluggish circulation. When a free-flowing, oxygenated bloodstream travels throughout your body, your trillions of cells and tissues become free of blockages and you are rewarded with a feeling of youthful health. You can experience this "reborn" feeling with the use of miracle power foods that can give you a dynamic circulation.

HOW FOODS BOOST YOUTHFUL CIRCULATION

Certain everyday foods and supplements have built-in natural substances that wash away the toxic wastes that otherwise impede your circulatory system. These foods have the gentle but thorough scrubbing ability to dislodge the glue-like encumbrances that interfere with a free-flowing circulation. Once these foods have cleansed the pathways, you can enjoy a form of regeneration through youthful (and youth-building) circulation.

Speedy Detoxification = Dynamic Circulation These miracle power foods aim directly at removing blockages from the pathways through which important nutrients must travel. These same foods actually widen the arteries and veins of your circulatory system to promote a better exchange of waste products and oxygen so that you can have a cleaner and more youthful metabolism. These miracle foods cleanse the pathways for a more vigorous transportation of wastes for elimination.

Swift Cleansing, Immediate Total Alertness   It is the enzymatic catalysts in these miracle foods that create swift cleansing. They also regenerate the damaged and broken capillaries almost at once. These are the smallest elements of your vascular unit. The exchange of oxygen for wastes takes place through the semipermeable walls of these capillaries. Constant breakdown of capillaries will reduce their filtering efficiency. These walls often become toxic-laden and this creates blockages which, in turn, can reduce the vital cleansing process that is so important in maintaining youthful health. Therefore, you need to have miracle foods available for (1) dispatching and dispersing accumulated wastes, and (2) repairing your capillaries so they are strong and able to function effectively as filters. With these miracle foods, you will enjoy swift cleansing and repair, and immediate total alertness.

ONE-DAY GRAPE JUICE FAST = FOREVER YOUNG CIRCULATION

Every ten days, plan to go on a grape juice fast for just one day. Take no foods, no other liquids, except for water. Throughout this entire day, drink unsweetened grape juice.

Cleanses, Rejuvenates, Exhilarates Circulation   The rich concentration of enzymes, combined with the high Vitamin C content, work swiftly to cleanse away accumulated wastes from the components that make up your circulatory network. The grape juice enzymes will stimulate gastric secretion and motility to boost this cleansing effect. The enzymes and the Vitamin C also create an antibacterial action that promotes a natural colonic cleansing which is then able to better discharge the waste products that might otherwise cause circulatory blockages.

Without the digestive competition of other foods and beverages, your enzymatic system is able to make full use of the grape juice nutrients to promote this cleansing reaction. You will feel rejuvenated as you enjoy a more exhilarating and sparklingly clean circulation.

One Day Works Lifetime Wonders Just one day (every ten days or so) can so supercharge your gastroenteric functions that you can experience the lifetime wonder of youthful circulation. Plan to enjoy this naturally sweet and speedily cleansing grape juice fast program regularly and you will be rewarded with a feeling of total youth.

Firms Up Skin, Enjoys Regularity, Doubles Energy

Bookkeeper Frank E.P. complained of feeling "clogged up." He had sagging skin, discomforting irregularity and a gradual loss of energy. As the days wore on, he became wearier and wearier. At times, the long debit-credit columns seemed to grow blurry before his bloodshot eyes. Frank E.P.'s work productivity declined. Confiding in his supervisor, he was told to visit the company physiologist. Tests showed that his circulation was being "choked" with blockages of wastes from end products of improperly metabolized foods. Frank E.P. was told to go on a simple one day grape juice fast every other week. He followed this amazingly simple program. He was doubly amazed when he felt energy rebounding. His skin became firm and smooth. He had restored regularity. He not only went through his balance sheet preparation speedily; he could work overtime with twice as much energy. He thanks this circulation-cleansing one day grape juice fast as the key to his feeling of "total rejuvenation."

"EARLY MORNING CIRCULATION BOOSTER"

The rate of circulation while you sleep is different from the day. Some days accumulation of wastes may act as blockages so that you just cannot get started in the morning. To help wash away these accumulations, boost your circulation with the use of four everyday miracle power foods in a dynamic combination.

HOW TO PREPARE BOOSTER

1 cup of fresh orange juice
1 teaspoon of brewer's yeast (from health store)
2 teaspoons of fortified powdered milk
1 egg

Blenderize all ingredients for just 20 seconds. Then sip slowly before you have breakfast.

Cleansing-Energizing Benefits: The invigorating Vitamin C of the orange juice combines with the powerful B-complex vitamins of the yeast; they boost the rich protein concentration of the milk and egg to create an almost "instantaneous" cell-scrubbing reaction. These same dynamic ingredients now surge through your circulatory system, sweeping away wastes, waking up your sluggish circulation, filling your bloodstream with throbbing vitality. Within 30 minutes after you finish this "Early Morning Circulation Booster," you will feel a revival of dynamic energy. This is the reward for having cleansed your circulatory system upon awakening.

Booster Gives Her Unlimited "Get Up and Go"

Homemaker Diane O'J. felt mounting responsibilities of home, local social affairs, and a part-time job taking such a toll that she just wanted to sleep all the time. She would wake up tired and remain so as she went through her daily chores—taking care of her family, carrying out her job. She walked with a stooped gait, and was slow with her reflexes. Often, her memory was vague. And she was only in her middle 40's. A sympathetic co-worker suggested she use the easily prepared "Early Morning Circulation Booster" that had been prescribed by a nutritionist for her own sluggishness. Diane O'J. tried it without delay, anxious to get out of her deepening slump. Within two days, she was completely refreshed. She enjoyed her many activities. She walked with a youthful bounce, had speedy reflexes, and enjoyed a sharp memory. The tasty booster had reversed her aging process and rewarded her with unlimited "get up and go." Life was so wonderful!

LIMIT (OR ELIMINATE) THESE CIRCULATION-BLOCKING FOODS

To help unblock and keep your circulation unblocked, be restrictive with these sets of "glue-like" foods that deposit heavy burdens of waste at vital checkpoints throughout your system.

- Whole milk, chocolate milk, malts, shakes, heavy cream.
- Luncheon meats, sausages, frankfurters, heavily marbled meats, poultry with skin, panfried or deep-fried (in fats) meats, poultry, commercially prepared meats, poultry with breading, gravies, sauces.

- Frozen or canned vegetables in a butter or cream sauce or deep fat-fried, or containing added salt and chemicals.
- Bread products (biscuits, muffins, pancakes, waffles, doughnuts) made with cream, whole milk, animal fats, chemicals.
- Coconut oil, cocoa butter or palm oil, hydrogenated or "hardened" vegetable shortening, meat drippings, suet or lard.
- Commercially prepared gravies or sauces. If homemade, avoid those containing large proportions of animal fats and salt or harsh seasonings.
- Ice cream, whipped cream, ice milk or frozen desserts containing previously named animal or "hard" fats.
- Chocolate, fudge, caramels, custard and puddings made with whole milk, commercial cakes, pies, cookies and mixes of unknown ingredients.
- Commercially fried foods such as potato chips and other deep-fried snacks which have been dunked in waste-causing fats.

Why These Are Harmful Foods   They are sources of hard fats and additives that leave thick deposits of sludge throughout your circulatory system. Continual intake of these waste-forming foods will cause a "pileup" of debris to form blockades. Your circulation is in risk of being narrowed down or choked off completely. This can take its toll in your cellular rejuvenation process. You need not assault your circulatory system with this food pollution. By simple limit or, better yet, elimination of certain foods, you can control waste accumulation and help give your circulation the free-flowing power it needs to help give you a feeling of improved youth.

THE CLOT-CLEANSING VITAMIN THAT MAY SAVE YOUR LIFE

When excess wastes are allowed to accumulate, they force the blood to form clots. These waste-filled clots become blockades in the bloodstream; that is, they block the free flow of circulating blood. Furthermore, these same wastes are glue-like in that they cause blood cells (called platelets) to stick together to form these dangerous clots.

Glue-Filled Platelets Are Life Risk   If allowed to accumulate, these platelets do more than just glue themselves together as a clot. They release granules containing a dangerous waste called adenosine diphosphate or ADP. This pollutant is a highly concentrated grain-like set of particles within the platelets. Once ADP is released, it spreads to make other platelets become glued together. *Danger:* They form clumps which block blood flow out of the vessel and this leads to a possible stroke. So you can see the danger to your life if you have an excess of these glue-filled platelets.

Vitamin B6 Is Super Cell Cleanser   This isolated member of the B-complex family (also called pyridoxine) blocks the action of ADP. It cleanses the cells and thereby controls the glue-like platelet aggregation. It dilutes this substance, promotes the washing away of it, and thereby guards against a life-threatening clot. It has super cell cleansing power.

The higher the pyridoxine levels you have available, the greater your protection against cellular pollution and the clot-causing ADP. Vitamin B6 or pyridoxine helps cleanse your cells and gives you a more vigorous and youthful circulation.

Sources of Cell-Cleansing Vitamin B6   Enjoy bananas; peanuts; tomatoes; all whole grain products such as breads, cereals, wheat germ, bran, and brewer's yeast. Include these foods in your menu for each day. Supplements are available at health stores.

By boosting your blood levels of Vitamin B6, you boost your cell cleansing powers and protect yourself against the threat of a blood clot choking away your breath of life.

Breathes Better, Looks Younger, Feels Revived in Eight Days

Shortness of breath and chronic fatigue sent Ned DiN. to his respiratory specialist. A few tests showed that he had a dangerously high level of glue-like platelet clumps. Their released ADP particles created circulatory blockages, the cause of his ill health. The specialist put him on a high Vitamin B6 program. Each day he was to use the wheat germ and bran as well as the other foods containing this cell cleanser. Ned DiN. started to breathe better almost at once.

Fatigue was gone and replaced with unusual vitality. He glowed with youthful health. Within eight days, he felt "eighty years younger," as he quipped, thanks to the cell-cleansing power of this amazing vitamin.

"TRIPLE CIRCULATION PICK-UP ELIXIR"

You can triple your circulation powers when you super-clean your cells with this tasty and invigorating elixir.

```
1 cup grapefruit juice
3 teaspoons fortified powdered milk
1 teaspoon wheat germ
1 teaspoon bran
½ banana
1 egg
```
Blenderize all ingredients for 30 seconds.

To Use: Drink one glass at noontime each day.

Internal Washing Benefits: The rich concentration of Vitamin C plus pectin (a powerful cell cleanser and rebuilder) activates the protein of the milk to join with the pyridoxine of the grains. With the minerals in the banana and the complete protein of the egg, they actually scour your circulatory system. This combination works together to propel these wastes right out of your system. The rich concentration of natural fruit sugars works to energize your circulatory system. In a short while, you feel a flow of vitality that makes you act with youthful vigor. Clean circulation adds up to this picked-up feeling.

The "Triple Circulation Pick-Up Elixir" does, in effect, triple the vigor of your circulation and give you that head-to-toe lively feeling to make you glad and healthy all over.

Instant Vigor with Elixir

Stooped shoulders, a hangdog expression and unrelieved fatigue so upset Olga B.Y., that she almost became a hermit. She could not keep up with people older than herself. Fortunately, she heard a radio interview with a nutritionist who told of the "Triple Circulation Pick-Up Elixir," and how it initiated internal washing to boost the energy powers of the circulatory system. Listening to it, Olga B.Y. decided to give it a try. Almost the same day, she could walk erectly, brighten up her face, and feel throbbing energy flowing through her body. Within three days she was so full of life she even went disco dancing. . . with folks much younger than herself. When she won a prize, she said her secret was "triple circulation" power. It had, indeed, picked her up and made her look and act alive again with instant vigor.

Unblock those waste deposits. Set your circulation free. Let oxygen transport energy-boosting nutrients and cell-repairing elements throughout your body. With the use of miracle power foods, you will experience dynamic circulation rejuvenation. Enjoy this restoration of total youth.

MAIN POINTS

1. Cleanse away circulation blockages with an occasional one-day grape juice fast. It made Frank E.P. become rejuvenated with the breath of life.

2. Wake up your sluggish responses with an "Early Morning Circulation Booster." It scrubs your cells and gives you powerful vigor. It gave fatigued Diane O'J. unlimited "get up and go."

3. Cut down on circulation-blocking foods as listed in this chapter.

4. Ned DiN. used Vitamin B6 (pyridoxine) as a super cell cleanser and enjoyed restored and revived circulation with youthful vitality in just eight days.

5. Olga B.Y. overcame her premature aging and chronic tired feeling with a tasty "Triple Circulation Pick-Up Elixir," within three days.

CHAPTER **10**

How to "Unlock" and "Release" Wastes for Freedom from "Aging Stiffness"

An accumulation of wastes that cling stubbornly to the multicellular components of your joints can be the underlying cause of your complaints of muscle stiffness. These leftover byproducts of internal combustion back up and block the free passage of oxygen and circulating blood. These wastes interfere with the nourishment of your joints and muscles. They choke your circulatory system at vital depots and create such blockades that you wince with pain if you have to reach for an object on a high shelf, or if you need to bend at the waist to look in a low shelf. This indicates that your cellular system has become heavily laden with these waste byproducts.

Daily Usage Causes Toxic Waste Backup   As you perform your daily chores, however mild or vigorous, you use your entire set of joints and muscles. To energize these segments, a biological reaction occurs. There is a transformation of adenosine triphosphate (ATP) into adenosine diphosphate (ADP). This gives you the energy to use your joints and muscles. In the meantime, this process also deposits a substance called *lactic acid*, which actually is a toxic waste. It exists only as part of the biological process of supplying energy and then leaves behind some refuse that needs to be eliminated. But it is this lactic acid that often tends to accumulate and create toxic waste backup.

WASH OUT LACTIC ACID FOR GREATER JOINT-MUSCLE FLEXIBILITY

To put more flexibility into your joints and muscles you must create an internal cleansing action that actually washes out the lactic acid blockages. In particular, you need to oxygenate your system so that the waste can (1) be largely eliminated, and (2) be transformed into glycogen, a prime energy source. It is oxygen that will perform this double-action body energizer, that is, rid your body of much of the lactic acid, and then create glycogen which gives you youthful flexibility in your joints and muscles.

THE FOOD THAT WASHES WASTES AND REJUVENATES JOINTS

Lecithin is a miracle food. Available as a supplement in granule form at most health stores, it performs a dynamic cleansing action that can give you youthful flexibility in a short time.

Contains Powerful Waste-Washer As a bland, water-soluble product made from de-fatted soybeans, lecithin contains a little-known substance called *acetylcholine*. This is a powerful waste-washer that can rejuvenate your body and provide you with superior joint-muscle flexibility almost as soon as it is consumed. Lecithin releases acetylcholine, which then triggers off the conversion of ATP to ADP. During this instantaneous process, the lecithin-distributed acetylcholine sweeps up lactic acid wastes, dilutes this sludge, and uses the energy-packed ADP to wash it right out of your body. Within minutes after you introduce this miracle food, lecithin, this waste-washing process takes place. That is why you will experience more flexibility in your joints and muscles so very rapidly. It is a super-cleanser and super-energizer because of this biological reaction.

Cleanses Brain, Liver, Bloodstream This food actually helps cleanse your brain because lecithin acetylcholine washes wastes from nerve cells to give you more reflex strength and better thinking ability. It also works to metabolize accumulated fat from your liver and guards against buildup of wastes that may lead to degeneration of this organ. Lecithin acetylcholine also acts as a guard in washing away fat that might otherwise accumulate in your bloodstream to be deposited in your arteries. So you can readily appreciate the dynamic overall cleansing power of lecithin.

HOW TO USE LECITHIN FOR SPEEDY JOINT-MUSCLE ENERGY

To correct the so-called "aging" of your joints and muscles, use lecithin daily to help wash away the lactic acid accumulations.

Basic Guidelines: Sprinkle several teaspoons of lecithin in soups, with your salads (fruit or vegetables), in baked goods, in juices. Add to your cereals, hot or cold. Stir into any dairy dish, such as yogurt. Take advantage of lecithin's emulsifying powers by adding the granules to gravies, sauces, dressings. Even small amounts of lecithin can improve the workability of the batter of any baking mixture, and boost the quality of the finished product. Yes, you can *eat and clean your body at the same time,* when lecithin is part of the recipe.

"INSTANT POWER POTION"

To a glass of fresh citrus juice, add two tablespoons of lecithin granules, a teaspoon of honey, one-half teaspoon of brewer's yeast. Blenderize for just 30 seconds. Drink slowly.

Speedy Energy   Within moments after swallowing, the Vitamin C of the juice invigorates the acetylcholine of the lecithin to wash away the lactic acid wastes from your joints and muscles. This combination is further energized by the concentrated minerals in the honey and the stimulation from the B-complex vitamins in the brewer's yeast. The reaction is an enormous internal scouring that occurs within minutes. Shortly thereafter, your cleansed joints and muscles will feel youthfully flexible. You will be able to move with the agility of a youngster. That is the power of this dynamic food combination.

Triple Energy with Easy Program   To experience triple energy, just drink this "Instant Power Potion" three times a day. After breakfast, at noontime, then in the early evening. You will be scrubbing away lactic acid throughout the day. You will also be transforming the waste substance, ATP, into the energy-producing ADP. This cleansing-energizing process will give you three-fold vitality throughout the day. Your joints and muscles will be flexible and capable of fulfilling your daily chores.

From "Too Tired" to "Too Active" in Three Days

No matter what George E. had to do, he was always "too tired." His wife complained that work piled up because he just could not muster enough strength to do even simple tasks. He complained his joints were stiff. His muscles ached if he carried a small bundle. At work as a factory foreman he became neglectful, let errors creep by because his body was always so "tight" that he could not make the necessary corrections. A neuromuscular physician diagnosed his problem as "cement-like" sludge accumulating on his joints and muscles. An excess of lactic acid was responsible for his chronic muscular fatigue. He suggested the "Instant Power Potion," three times daily. George E. began at once. Immediately, he felt his joints and muscles becoming loosened up. Within two days, he could do a good day's work at the factory and many chores at home at night. By the end of the third day, his "too tired" feeling was gone. His co-workers and wife chided him for being "too active." The washing away of constricting and choking wastes had given him youthful flexibility.

HOW TO VENTILATE YOUR JOINTS
FOR GREATER MOBILITY

Simple body motions or exercises that you perform during your daily routine can send a stream of waste-washing oxygen throughout your body. In moments the lactic acid is dispelled, the sludge byproducts of adenosine triphosphate (ATP) are washed away, and your entire circulatory system becomes refreshed. Just fit these easy (and fun) exercises into your schedule and be rewarded with greater mobility.

1. A railing is required for use as a dance bar. Grab onto the bar and alternately kick your legs out behind you. Now turn and lift your legs out to the side, first facing the front of the room, then the back. Just five minutes daily helps boost the cleansing process that will limber up your tight muscles.

2. After your bath, sit on the tub's edge. Stretch both arms in all directions. When drying yourself, hold the towel up around the back of your neck; move your arms from side to side, twisting your body from left to right as you dry off. This movement will exhilarate your entire body.

3. When in a warm bath, lift your legs and stretch your toes. The comfortable heat of the bath will unlock sludge and prepare it for evaporation while your taut muscles become more flexible.

4. When sweeping the floor (not an enjoyable task, but it can be made beneficial), use the broom as a support. Stretch your right leg backwards. Then reverse and stretch your left leg backwards. Keep doing this as you sweep—it oxygenates your system and also makes sweeping less of a tedious chore.

5. Frequently, rise up and down on your toes. The accelerated breathing will oxygenate your circulatory system and ventilate your joints and muscles to promote flexibility.

With daily use of these body movements, you will give your joints and muscles a form of daily scrubbing that will make you feel flexible all over.

GARLIC: DYNAMIC WASTE-WATCHER

Garlic contains an anti-oxidant substance that acts as more than a waste-watcher—it's a waste-washer, too. The dynamic anti-oxidant power means that it is able to swoop down on wastes, such as peroxides, toxins, free radicals (bits and scraps from incomplete metabolism), and keep them from accumulating to excess. The very presence of garlic with its mitogenetic radiation factor means that wastes do not remain for long in your joint-muscle system. Garlic will uproot these ache- and pain-causing wastes and prepare them for elimination. Garlic, therefore, acts as a guard to protect your body against waste overload.

Eat Garlic Daily Just two or three well-chewed cloves daily will make these waste-watching elements available and help keep your cells clean. This easy and tasty program can help you enjoy a more flexible range of your joints and muscles.

Garlic Chewing Frees Joints from Stiffness

Waitress Dolores LaF. was told that her job was in jeopardy because she could hardly carry even moderately heavy trays of food to the restaurant customers. Even having to wipe off a table made her wince with pain because of her limited joint range; tears involuntarily came down her face, which was hardly an appetizing sight for customers. Complaining to a produce deliveryman, she was told that he, too, suffered from joint stiffness to the point where he doubled up in pain. Then he heard of garlic as a European remedy for this muscular problem, and began to chew it daily. He regained full use of his arms and legs. Dolores LaF. decided to try it. She also chewed much parsley, sometimes a cinnamon stick (in private) to protect against offending anyone. Within two days, the tightness in her muscles vanished. Within four days, she could carry a heavier than usual tray with the greatest of ease. She could wash and clean with full joint-muscle range. Garlic had cleansed away the sediment that caused the stiffness. She could even work overtime with no complaints!

HOW TO STEAM WASTES OUT OF YOUR JOINTS

Luxuriate in a bath filled with comfortably warm water. It should be warm enough so that you perspire. This creates an outpouring of melted-down joint-muscle wastes that are released through the steam-opened pores. Just 30 minutes will help steam most of the blockage-forming wastes out of your body. You'll emerge from the tub with more flexible joints and more resilient muscles.

Remove the "rust" from your joints and muscles with corrective nutrition, simple exercises, and steaming and you will enjoy freedom from "aging stiffness."

SUMMARY

1. Regular daily usage of joints and muscles will cause lactic acid waste backup that blocks free joint-muscle flexibility.
2. Lecithin helps wash such wastes out of your system and restores youthful movement to your limbs.
3. George E. went from "too tired" to "too active" in three days with the help of the cleansing benefit of the tasty "Instant Power Potion."

4. Dolores LaF. ended her agonizing joint-muscle stiffness with the help of super-cleansing garlic.
5. Steam wastes out of your joints with a comfortable 30-minute warm water tub immersion.

CHAPTER 11

Cleanse Your Organs for Total Revitalization

Wash away wastes and debris from your vital organs and experience total revitalization from head to toe. With clean organs, you will be able to see and hear better, enjoy a more youthful metabolism, and feel the joy of everyday living. When these organs are washed free of accumulated wastes, they function at maximum efficiency so that you are rewarded with strong reflexes and the look and feel of overall youth. An added bonus of cleansed organs is the freedom from discomfort, aches, disorders, and toxic-caused ailments.

LESS SUGAR + LESS STRAIN = STRONGER EYESIGHT[1]

"You can improve your eyesight, especially your nearsightedness, by cutting down your intake of sugar (sources of wastes) and reducing prolonged strain," said optometrist Ben C. Lane, in a talk before the annual meeting of the Optical Society of America. "In addition, a mineral imbalance of chromium and calcium in the body can also create conditions that lead to possible nearsightedness."

Sugar Wastes Are Cause of Visual Problems Based on laboratory tests, Dr. Lane says that the intake of sugar, along with other

---

[1]*Natural Health Bulletin,* Delta Group, 1101D State Road, Princeton, N.J., 08540, Feb. 11, 1980 and June 30, 1980. Available by subscription.

refined carbohydrates, may cause a depletion of the body's store of chromium. "Sugar also forces the body to use its supplies of B-complex vitamins that are needed to regulate fluid pressure in the eye." Furthermore, "Folks with worsening nearsightedness consume relatively more sugar and other refined carbohydrates than those with unchanging eyesight." *Suggestion:* Avoid sugar in any form. Eliminate refined carbohydrates from your diet. Both foods deposit toxic waste refuse in your circulatory system and this appears to drain out valuable sight-saving vitamins and chromium.

Strain Causes Visual Weakness   Repeated, unrelieved eyestrain from excessive, close-up visual work, says Dr. Lane, "may lead to an increase in eye fluid pressure which results in nearsightedness. If the close-up work is done day after day for more than a couple of weeks, fluid pressure increases and the eye starts to react." This causes visual weakness; specifically the problem of nearsightedness.

Mineral Deficiency Is Probable Cause   Hair samples showed that folks with worsening nearsightedness have a "washing out" of calcium from the body. Dr. Lane says, "One effect of eating too much 'overcooked protein' is the loss of important B-complex vitamins which, in turn, leads to a calcium loss." Make this simple adjustment: switch to more fresh foods, whole grains, lean meats or fish which are cooked to tenderness, but not to excess which increases deposition of wastes. These, in turn, tend to dissolve the valuable vitamins and calcium which are needed to maintain healthy eyesight.

Toxemia: Root of Nearsightedness   An overloading of toxic wastes can contribute to nearsightedness, also known as myopia. The toxemia overload causes a change in the outward or convex curvature of the eye lens. *Explanation:* Normal eye muscles change the lens curvature constantly as you focus on objects at different distances. To focus on a nearby object, eye muscles elongate the eyeball to increase this curvature to enable light from nearby objects to focus on the retina. *Problem:* An accumulation of wastes creates an increased convexity which builds up more fluid pressure in the eye. *Washing Plan:* Dr. Lane theorizes that if this fluid pressure could be regulated through elimination of waste-causing sugar and the easing of visual and muscular strain, then nearsightedness might be controlled and, hopefully, corrected. By eliminating sugar, you create a washing reaction that can give you healthier eyesight.

LESS COOKING = LESS INTERNAL WASTES

Overcooking Is Problem   Says Dr. Lane, "The 'washing out' of calcium generally appears to be caused not by insufficient calcium intake, but rather by mishandling of dietary calcium as a result of excessive intake of overcooked protein.

"This overcooking turns wholesome protein into a deficit-inducing food. This also depletes vitamins, including B6, which are essential to the utilization of both the protein and the protein-bound calcium. This calcium mishandling does not itself increase the inner eye pressure, but allows the white of the eye (sclera) to become more stretchable when the effects of chromium depletion or Vitamin C depletion elevate the intraocular pressure."

Say No to Sugar and Refined Carbohydrates   To improve the sight organs, Dr. Lane advises, "We need to avoid eating sugar and refined carbohydrates which deplete the body reserves of chromium and vitamins, thereby preventing normal regulation of intraocular pressure."

Cleaner Eyes for Better Vision   "Preventive measures in eye care may help prevent many people from having to wear strong glasses and strong contact lens prescriptions. But we should see more young people using special, quite low in power "reading glasses" to reduce the accommodative eye-focusing demands for the close work of today's culture. Public education on myopia and nutrition in general," concludes Dr. Lane, "should result in a turnaround in sugar consumption and reduced size of protein portions." This would create cleaner visual organs and better eyesight.

Reverses Deteriorating Eyesight in 11 Days on Easy Program

As a machinist, Oscar T. felt that his job was being jeopardized by his worsening eyesight. He had to squint even at close range. His eyeglasses became stronger and stronger while his sight became weaker and weaker. At times, he required help from a co-worker who complained that he wasn't Oscar's seeing eye dog! This cutting remark brought Oscar T. to his ophthalmologist for help. Tests were made and a problem of waste-clogging was identified. Also, his bloodstream showed an excessive sugar overload, as well as refuse wastes from refined carbohydrates. A mineral deficiency was also detected. Oscar T. was put on an easy program of no sugar in any form and no refined carbohydrates. He had to boost his intake of calcium and chromium and eat less overcooked protein foods, too. Almost at once, his vision became sharper. Within one week, Oscar T. could decipher tool markings without his too-strong glasses. By the eleventh day, he required very weak glasses and could read with the acuity of a young person. He could read books, road signs, and see movies without the need for eyeglasses. The simple program outlined by his ophthalmologist had reversed his deteriorating eye-sight within this short span of time. He can now remark that his restored vision is stronger than a seeing eye dog's!

HOW VITAMIN C + BIOFLAVONOIDS WASH AWAY CATARACT DEBRIS

These two above-mentioned vitamins exert a powerful cleansing reaction that will help wash away the grainy substances that lead to the formation of cataracts. In this condition, waste accumulation causes an increasing opacity and threat of vision loss; it is similar to a window getting frosted by cold until only the strongest light can be seen through it. To help protect against this thief of sight, wash away the debris with the use of Vitamin C and bioflavonoids.

Vitamin C Is Protective Cleanser   A high concentration of this vitamin helps cleanse away debris in the lens of the eye and in the fluid directly in front of it (between lens and cornea). Vitamin C in the aqueous humor (as the fluid is called) acts as a protective cleanser and guards against toxic buildup that may cause cataracts. Have Vitamin C available and you have good protection against sight deterioration.

Bioflavonoids Block Waste Corrosion   A class of nutrients that complement the action of Vitamin C are bioflavonoids ,which block the action of a waste corrosion substance called *aldose reductase*. This substance irritates certain components of your eyes and brings about a corrosion that could predispose to cataracts. Bioflavonoids will dilute the potentially harmful wastes of *aldose reductase*, and keep it washed out of your aqueous humor fluid. You can protect yourself against cataracts with regular intake of bioflavonoids.

Everyday Sources of Vitamin C, Bioflavonoids Citrus fruits (oranges, grapefruits, tangerines, lemons, limes, papaya, strawberries, cantaloupe, tomato, broccoli, green peppers, raw leafy greens. *Caution:* Vitamin C is water-soluble and is not stored in your body. Take in a good supply of these foods and their juices daily. Bioflavonoids are found in highly concentrated form in the stringy portions near the rinds of your citrus fruits. Plan to eat (yes, eat!) these strings when you eat the fruits. You'll be giving your metabolism the needed bioflavonoids that wash away debris from your aqueous humor, and thus safeguard your vision. Supplements are available at health stores, too.

Sight-Saving Tonic Washes Away Cataracts

Schoolteacher Minna S. was troubled with dimming vision. Blackboard writings became blurred. Identifying pupils was confusing. Fearing the problem of cataracts, she was examined by a sight specialist who said that tests showed a deposit of wastes in her aqueous humor fluid. These wastes were clouding her vision and threatening to erode her delicate eye segments. He suggested she use a "Sight-Saving Tonic" that would introduce super-cleansing Vitamin C and bioflavonoids into her system. These cleansers would wash away debris and give her sparkling visual fluid. They would also block and eliminate *aldose reductase*, the corrosive waste that could create cataracts. Minna S. tried the tonic. Within four days, she could see better. Writing on the blackboard was sharp. At the end of six days, she had excellent vision. Gone was the threat of cataracts.

How to Prepare "Sight-Saving Tonic" Use a variety of citrus fruits, especially grapefruit and tangerine. Remove the peels but retain the white, string-like membrane. Juice the fruits in an electric extractor or a blender. This tonic is a powerhouse of valuable bioflavonoids. Drink three glasses of this "Sight-Saving Tonic" daily.

Washes Debris, Boosts Sight Strength Within moments after swallowing the tonic, the rich concentration of Vitamin C, along with the bioflavonoids unite to create a super-washing of visual debris. They further nourish the cells and tissues of your eyes and improve power of vision. They cleanse your aqueous humor fluid so it sparkles with clean health. You see with sparkling clarity, too. It is a tasty, refreshing, and sight-strengthening tonic that works swiftly.

BETTER HEARING WITH CLEANER EARS

Hearing loss is gradual. Wastes accumulate within your auditory segments, clinging together and slowly choking off the transfer of sounds. The end result could be impaired hearing. To protect against this toxic waste buildup, it is important to take advantage of home programs that clean away such debris. To understand the effectiveness of this ear-washing program, you must become familiar with the basics about your hearing apparatus.

How Do You Hear?   Your ear is made up of three separate parts.

1. *Visible Outer Ear.* A trumpet-shaped organ with a funnel or duct that reaches into your ear drum. This is a thin, tautly stretched membrane which vibrates when struck by sound waves.

2. *Middle Ear.* On the opposite side of this membrane is your middle ear, made up of three small bones shaped like a hammer, anvil and a stirrup. When sound waves make the ear drum vibrate, this sound is transported across the three small bones and then into the fluid of your inner ear.

3. *Inner Ear.* Here are situated tiny, electrically charged hairs that bend and flex in response to noise and carry an electric-like current to the nerve of hearing. Your inner ear also is the site of a fluid that bathes these hairs and keeps them clean and alert. These microscopic hairs move back and forth, conducting the sound to the hearing nerve which then transmits it electrically to your brain.

Clean Membrane = Sharper Hearing   When your inner ear is kept washed of debris, it receives more vibrations through the cleaner membrane. Therefore, you should be able to hear sound frequencies of about 25,000 cycles per second. This enables you to hear with youthful acuity. It is when debris covers your membrane, when wastes clog up your inner ear fluids and turn them into waste puddles, that you begin to suffer hearing loss. Fewer and fewer cycles per second are heard and you do not hear ordinary conversation as well as you should. To correct this condition, cleanse away the debris that is clogging up your ear membrane and fluids.

HOW TO CLEANSE AND ENERGIZE YOUR EARS FOR SUPER-HEARING

A diet that is high in refined carbohydrates (sugars and starches) causes a speedy jump in your blood sugar. Moments thereafter, the blood sugar drops down as the refined sweets are metabolized. This causes and up-and-down insulin "yank," as it is called. It has its repercussions on your hearing.

Problem: Your inner ear has one of the highest needs for energy, as compared to other organs. An up-and-down blood sugar yank means that excessive amounts of wastes or "fallout" from refined foods are deposited on your membrane and in your fluids, and left there as there is a drop in blood sugar. A serious problem here is that such a shift causes a constriction of the highly sensitive vascular network in your ears. Your ears become "energy-starved." Oxygen is choked off, and nutrients cannot get to your ears; circulation also becomes blocked. Wastes are allowed to build up, which cannot be washed away. Your hearing starts to deteriorate.

Speedy Solution Eliminate all refined, processed and chemically treated foods. Avoid any refined carbohydrate foods. Boost your intake of fresh fruits, vegetables, whole grains, lean meat products.

Benefits: These foods are prime sources of Vitamin A, needed to nourish and cleanse the sensory receptor cells of the inner ears. They contain the B-complex vitamins that play an important role in a balanced blood sugar metabolism; they also cleanse the nerves of your hearing components. The foods contain Vitamin C, which scrubs away wastes, cleanses the membrane and also washes debris from the fluids in your inner ear and then scrubs clean the important microscopic hairs.

Within moments, hearing becomes improved and you enjoy better sound transmission, so that you no longer miss words or have to cup your ear to listen to normal conversational levels. Cleanse your hearing from *within* on this easy program and you speedily energize your ears for super-hearing from *without*.

THE LOW-FAT WAY TO IMPROVED HEARING

Reduce intake of hard animal fats. These cause red blood cells to become glued together, thus choking off the flow of oxygen to your inner ears. These blood levels of fats attract wastes and continue to grow so that blockages are erected to interfere with youthful hearing processes. You need to make a simple dietary change.

More Vegetable Fats for Better Hearing   Increase intake of free-flowing oils and non-hydrogenated fats (those that are liquid at room temperature). To control levels of fats in your bloodstream, restrict intake of any hard animal fats. You'll have clean red blood cells and improved hearing, too.

From "Nearly Deaf" to "Total Hearing" in 16 Days

As a sales manager, Benedict U. had to be a good listener as much as a good talker. So when he began to "miss" words or, worse, "misunderstand" what customers and supervisors said, he became worried. Gradually, his hearing diminished until he feared something worse than job loss—isolation from the world! He was examined by an audiologist (hearing specialist) who found that an overlayer of waste material had caused a clogging of his hearing apparatus. Too many hard fats had glued together his red blood cells. Too many refined foods caused an overflow of such toxic debris that his hearing was "choked" off. Benedict U. was put on a program of natural and low-fat foods. Within one week, his hearing improved. By the end of 16 days, he had conquered the spectre of being "nearly deaf" and enjoyed "total hearing." His cleansed hearing components made sound transmission as clear as that of a youngster's.

KEEP YOUR KIDNEYS CLEAN FOR INTERNAL REJUVENATION

Your kidneys are your body's filter plant, through which over 150 quarts of fluid pass daily. These two large organs in the small of your back filter your bloodstream and remove impurities.

Each kidney consists of a million tiny filters. Their task is to strain waste products out of your blood, dilute them in water and then excrete them in your urine. Blood enters one end of each tiny kidney tube and is propelled out through the other (smaller) end. This should be an effective filtering process, but if wastes are allowed to accumulate, then the blood becomes clogged and the risk of uremic poisoning presents itself. You can readily appreciate the value of having clean kidneys.

Simple Water Drinking Washes Away Kidney Debris Accumulated debris may cling together to form kidney stones. These are crystallized bits of wastes that back up in the kidneys. Most kidney stones consist of urates, phosphates, oxalates and other wastes that are improperly broken down or washed away. To protect against this accumulation, simple water drinking is a helpful method of kidney washing.

Washes, Cleanses, Rejuvenates The water you drink becomes part of your bloodstream and then is able to wash away waste products, cleanse your delicate kidney filters, and rejuvenate your kidney tubes. The same water is able to dilute the small, irritating, burr-like clumps that hook together and threaten to form into kidney stones. You become rejuvenated through drinking healthy water.

Daily quaffing of fresh water will also regulate your temperature, lubricate your joints and muscles, improve digestion, and facilitate the washing out of wastes from your entire body as well as your kidneys. It is the refreshing, rejuvenating way to have healthy organs.

Drinks Away Kidney Wastes in Short Time

Improper elimination of waste made Brenda O'R. feel sluggish. At times she was troubled with a sour stomach and a disposition to match! Her internist said she was "dehydrated" because she just neglected to consume enough water daily. She was diagnosed as having kidney wastes that could clump together and form stones and would require surgery. Anxious to avoid the knife, she followed the internist's amazingly simple program, which was to drink 6 to 8 glasses of water daily. Immediately, Brenda O'R. felt a clearing up of her sluggishness. In four days, she felt alert, more energetic. In six days, she was cheerful in body, mind, and attitude. Her internist confirmed her hopes. The wastes had actually been washed away. She was saved from the threat of surgical removal of kidney stones . . . thanks to drinking water!

THE BERRY JUICE THAT DISSOLVES KIDNEY GRAVEL

Cranberry juice is a prime source of Vitamin C, along with a natural fruit acid that is reportedly able to dissolve gravel in the kidneys and prepare it for speedy elimination.

The acid soil of New England which nurtures and nourishes the cranberry, gives to it the same strong scouring power that creates this cleansing action.

Drink Cranberry Juice Just two or three glasses of cranberry juice weekly will deliver a highly concentrated and potent acid to dissolve the gravel. *Cleansing Benefit:* The rich Vitamin C uses the cranberry acid to break up oxalate clumps and facilitate their removal through waste channels. It's the tasty and refreshing way to keep your kidneys clean and your body in youthful shape, too.

WASHING YOUR LIVER FOR TOTAL HEALTH

Your liver (largest body organ) performs many functions essential to your life. Therefore, if you keep it washed, you can then enjoy total health.

Located behind the lower ribs on the right side of your abdomen, your liver weighs about three pounds and is roughly the size of a football.

Functions: This master organ is responsible for removing from your blood both ingested and internally produced toxic wastes. Your liver converts them into a form that is easily eliminated. In essence, your liver is your body's refinery as it detoxifies and excretes substances that otherwise would be poisonous. It also makes bile, a fluid which is essential for digestion. It is involved in all of these processes which influence your levels of health. So a healthy liver can give you a healthy and vigorous life.

Waste Backup Leads to Liver Distress Waste accumulation hampers proper filtering by your liver and leads to such problems as skin discoloration (sometimes called jaundice), cirrhosis (scarring), abdominal swelling, fatigue, nausea. These symptoms suggest that the waste needs to be removed. At the same time, liver regeneration is needed so this master organ can bounce back with vitality to promote improved health.

Guidelines for Keeping Your Liver Clean   Protect your liver against pollution with these guidelines. Avoid all forms of salt, sugar and irritating seasonings. Avoid white flour products, commercial cereals, processed or artificially preserved soft drinks, alcohol, tobacco, fatty and fried foods, rancid oils.

At the same time, be sure to enjoy lots of exercise, fresh air and rest. These will help improve the health of your liver and your entire body. You'll feel refreshed and cleansed and made all over again, thanks to a washed liver.

HOW TO KEEP YOUR GALL BLADDER IN TIPTOP CONDITION

A part of your liver, your gall bladder is a small pear-shaped reservoir for a bitter fluid called bile which is needed to emulsify and digest fat in your intestine. Between meals, any bile that is not needed immediately is stored in your gall bladder. When food is ingested and prepared for assimilation, a tube from your gall bladder opens so that this digestive bile is able to pour into your intestine to metabolize the food. A problem often occurs if your bladder develops defects in function. It means that fragments of improperly digested food causes waste accumulation.

Wastes Form into Gallstones   When accumulated wastes crystallize in the bladder, they tend to form stones that vary in size from small pebbles to as large as golf balls. Sometimes, these stones get stuck in the bile ducts leading from the bladder to the duodenum (first part of small intestine). The bladder and bile ducts then try to push the stones out by muscular contractions. This can cause attacks of excruciating abdominal pain. Blockage of the ducts by stones also prevents flow of bile into the intestines. Bile then backs up into the bloodstream, causing jaundice. This is the obvious symptom of this waste backup.

THE FOOD THAT HELPS WASH AWAY
GALL BLADDER WASTES

Taken from soybeans, lecithin helps promote a bladder-scrubbing action that may well wash away stone-forming wastes. Lecithin is able to break down the precipitated cholesterol that is often part of the painful gallstones. Lecithin causes the manufacture of cholic acid, a natural scrubbing substance found in bile. Lecithin will then prompt this cholic acid to saturate the precipitated cholesterol crystals and break them down and help in their dissolution.

Lecithin is also a source of phospholipids which prevents cholesterol fats from clumping together. It works to break down these accumulations and free the bladder from the risk of glue-like encumbrances. Lecithin may well be the key to washing away gall bladder wastes.

Easy Ways to Use Sprinkle one teaspoon daily of granulated lecithin over salads; add to soups, stews, casseroles, baked goods. Or just add to a vegetable juice, stir vigorously (or blenderize) and drink slowly.

PLAIN WATER HELPS WASH AWAY BLADDER CRYSTALS

Drinking up to six glasses of plain water daily will help liquefy the crystals, provide a medium in which the grit can be washed right out of your eliminative channels.

Throughout the day, drink this important source of organ cleansing. Water helps keep your entire body as clean and sparkling fresh as itself.

Crystals Break Up, Wash Out of Body

Middle-aged Carole L. feared she would follow in the footsteps of her older sisters who underwent gall bladder removal. She felt frequent spasms, and was concerned with her sagging skin, dull complexion and discomfort after eating ordinary meals. She discussed it with her preventive-oriented physician, who suggested she follow a lecithin plan and also drink at least six glasses of water daily. Carole L. followed the program. Almost at once, the spasms and discomfort ended. Soon, her skin perked up. She was later examined and found to be out of any danger of stone formation. Carole L. had actually broken up (thanks to lecithin) and washed out (thanks to plain water) the accumulated wastes in a matter of less than two weeks.

Controlling Bladder Pollution Follow the general guidelines as outlined throughout this book, but to protect your bladder against stone-forming pollution, ease up or eliminate intake of any product containing salt, sugar, or white flour. Avoid hard animal fats as much as possible. Boost intake of fresh fruits, vegetables, whole grains, nuts, seeds, polyunsaturated free-flowing oils. Drink lots of water and freshly prepared juices. With these programs, you can help protect your bladder against the accumulation of wastes that may then form into pain-causing stones.

You can enjoy a feeling of total rejuvenation when you have sparkling clean internal organs. Free them of debris and glue-like wastes, and you will then know what a wonderful joy life can be.

IN REVIEW

1. Wash away wastes and improve your eyesight on a sugar-free and refined carbohydrate-free program as recommended by one doctor.
2. Oscar T. reversed his deteriorating eyesight in 11 days on a simple cleansing program.
3. Vitamin C + bioflavonoids wash away cataract-forming debris.
4. Schoolteacher Minna S. used the tasty "Sight-Saving Tonic" to save her eyes from surgery.
5. Sharpen your hearing on an improved nutritional program. It calls for low animal fats for cleaner ears and better hearing.
6. Benedict U. went from "nearly deaf" to "total hearing" in just about two weeks on the simple food program.
7. Brenda O'R. was able to wash and cleanse her kidneys on an easy water drinking plan.
8. Cranberry juice is a tasty way to help dissolve kidney gravel.

9. Lecithin helps cleanse your bladder and keep it in tiptop condition. Water also helps wash away bladder crystal wastes.

10. Carole L. followed a lecithin and water plan that ended her bladder distress.

CHAPTER *12*

How to Cleanse Your Bloodstream and Enrich Your Entire Body

The cleaner your bloodstream, the healthier your body. When you realize that every part of your body is bathed, washed, nourished, and oxygenated by your bloodstream constantly, you will understand the importance of having a clean "river of life." You need to have rich red blood cells that are able to deposit essential nutrients on all your vital organs, as well as your trillions of tissues. This is your very foundation of inner rejuvenation. You can free yourself from internal pollution with a clean bloodstream.

Continuous Process Calls for Rich Blood   Your circulatory system is responsible for: the uninterrupted delivery of oxygenated blood and its nutrients to your trillions of tissue cells; their exchange for waste products of metabolism; and the transportation of wastes to points of elimination. Hardly any other body system has such a great responsibility as your circulatory system because, without a supply of clean, oxygenated blood, your tissues and cells would soon die. To keep them more than just alive, but throbbing with youthful vitality, you need to have rich and very clean blood.

Sediment in Blood Causes Ill Health   As blood flows through your circulatory system, it picks up waste products left through oxidation and is responsible for their elimination. During this process, the waste products are passed through the microscopically thin walls of your capillaries (tiny cells). It is inevitable that some sediment remains behind. If there is a brief spell of sluggish-

125

ness, more waste tends to remain in the bloodstream instead of being discharged through your capillaries. Incomplete metabolism will also leave fragments and bits of refuse still in your bloodstream. If allowed to build up, such sediment can cause a choking off of your free-flowing blood circulation and pave the way to ill health. You need to keep your blood clean with simple, effective home washing programs. Let's see how you can do this without any delay.

THE EVERYDAY FOOD THAT CREATES A SPARKLING CLEAN BLOODSTREAM

Remove the most stubborn sludge deposits from your blood and be rewarded with a sparkling clean bloodstream with the use of a tangy everyday food. *Garlic.* This amazing food is able to initiate the synthesis, or the breakdown, of the waste substances that cling to your red and white blood cells. Garlic is then able to dissolve these wastes and propel them toward your eliminative channels. It becomes a powerful blood cleanser.

Two Powerful Blood Cleansing Substances in Garlic Almost immediately after you consume garlic, your digestive system metabolizes two of its most powerful cleansers. They are allylpropyldisulfide and diallyldisulfide. In combination, they swirl through your circulatory system, acting like magnets in attracting wastes, uprooting these sludge deposits, breaking down stubborn clumps, and speedily washing them right out of your body. This super-cleansing action occurs almost within minutes after you have consumed garlic. This everyday food is a miracle blood washer.

One Clove a Day Keeps Your Bloodstream Clean You may enjoy more than this amount, of course, but the minimum is just one clove a day of this powerful blood cleanser. You may add a finely chopped garlic clove to a plate of raw vegetables. You could also have garlic juice. Use a garlic press (at most health stores or housewares outlets) and squeeze several drops of juice from one or two cloves into a glass of freshly prepared vegetable juice. Just a few drops of garlic juice will do the trick. Stir vigorously and drink before your main meal. You could also add a few chopped cloves to a stew or soup or casserole or any baked dish. Just aim for at least one clove a day and you will be introducing a powerful "dirt magnet" into your bloodstream that will gather up the sludge and then whirl it right out of your body. A cleaner bloodstream will be your reward.

Corrects Cold Hands, Feet, Constant Chills in Two Days

Marcia J.H. had to wear sweaters and gloves in the warmest weather. As a computer operator, she complained of cold working conditions even when the heat was turned on at top levels. Marcia J.H. shivered even if she sat in the warm sun. A company registered nurse took some tests and said that Marcia had "unclean blood," which sounded as unpleasant as it felt! The nurse suggested she consume at least two garlic cloves daily with her regular meals to detoxify her sludge-filled blood. Because of toxic waste blockages, her bloodstream was choked off to the point where it could not provide warming oxygenated nourishment to her vital organs and cells. This was the root cause of her icy feeling even in warm weather.

Marcia J.H. followed the program. Immediately, she enjoyed a throbbing vitality. In two days, she was so warm, she glowed with a radiant complexion, and discarded her sweater and gloves. She even complained that the computer section was too warm! Garlic had warmed her body by cleansing her bloodstream in just two days.

HOW TO WASH AND "IRON" YOUR BLOOD CELLS FOR SUPER HEALTH

Put more life into your body with washed and "ironed" blood cells. This does not refer to any laundering iron. It means a "cell washing" first and then a "cell nourishing" second with the use of *iron*, the amazing nutrient. It has the power to invigorate your blood cells and give you the look and feel of super health. You can "wash out" and "iron-nourish" your blood cells in a simple two-part program. Here's how.

First: Cell-Washing Uproot the accumulated blood sediment and prepare it for elimination by opening your skin pores and steaming out these wastes. You do this in a simple and refreshing *contrast bath*. It takes just 20 minutes and gives you a feeling of lifetime youthfulness by cleaning your bloodstream. Follow these easy steps.

1. Fill your bathtub with water warm enough to create clouds of steam. It should be comfortable, but not burning, of course.

2. Immerse yourself. Luxuriate in the steaming warmth for about 15 minutes. You should perspire. This indicates the uprooted sediment is being washed out of your blood and body cells.

3. Let the water run out of the tub. Now stand up. (Careful! Hold on to a bar to avoid skidding.) Turn on a needle-spray *cool* shower. It should give you a pleasant (not hurtful) sting. This washes away your steamed-out sediment. The cool water closes your pores so you are protected against incoming pollutants. Less than three minutes of this contrasting cool shower is all you need.

4. Step on a non-skid bath mat. Dry yourself with a rough towel. You have helped steam out impurities and will be rewarded with a more invigorated bloodstream.

Second: Cell-Ironing   Your second step of this two-part "wash and iron" blood cell program calls for nutrition. You need to feed the breath of life to your cells by supplying them with *iron*. This nutrient is needed to help produce *hemoglobin,* the red coloring matter of your cells. Iron also increases and invigorates the formation of your white blood cells. Called *leukocytes,* they are a bit larger than the red ones. They have the lifesaving power of destroying toxic substances. But these white blood cells change all the time. They wear out, break down, disintegrate. If not replaced, they create a shortage which means that the sediment and wastes are accumulating. If improperly cleansed, these wastes stick together and create blockages which interfere with a free-flowing blood circulation. To boost the vigor and restoration of leukocytes or white cells that cleanse wastes, feed them iron!

Here is a cell-ironing (or iron-feeding) program that works:

1. Boost intake of these high iron-containing foods: liver, fish, whole grain cereals and breads, dark leafy green vegetables, sun-dried fruits such as apricots, raisins, brewer's yeast.

2. Combine iron foods together with a Vitamin C food. The iron is better absorbed when it is energized with the presence of Vitamin C *at the same time.* This is a booster iron-feeding technique

that will give an exhilarating rejuvenation to your white cells. Within moments, these foods scour your bloodstream and cleanse away debris to make you feel warm and alive all over. This combination works almost immediately and is tasty, too.

3. Take one to three tablespoons of desiccated liver (from health store) with any favorite fruit or vegetable juice daily. This gives you a high concentration of iron (without the fat present in the whole meat product) *together* with Vitamin C. This acts as a dynamic energizer to your blood-cleansing white cells.

4. Daily, take the "C + Iron Tonic" to create an immediate regeneration of your trillions of waste-washing white blood cells. *To Prepare:* In a glass of fresh citrus fruit juice, add one tablespoon of desiccated liver and one-half teaspoon of brewer's yeast. Stir vigorously or blenderize for 30 seconds. Drink just one glass of this "C + Iron Tonic" daily before your main meal. It is a powerhouse of cell rejuvenation and blood cleansing.

Restored to Life with "C + Iron Tonic"

Jennifer W.M. was troubled with shortness of breath. Her hands trembled. Her eyes looked dull. She had that aged, wizened appearance that made her look much older than her formerly-young age of 45. Family and friends said she was aging rapidly. Jennifer W.M. was told to take iron foods and supplements. She did, but the benefit was negligible. Something was wrong. Her hematologist (blood specialist) diagnosed her condition as a scarcity of important blood-washing white cells. The iron in the foods she was consuming was not being fully absorbed because it lacked Vitamin C at the same time. He told her to take the "C + Iron Tonic" daily. This *combination* would revitalize her system and the iron would be absorbed fully to give her white cells the ability to scour and cleanse her bloodstream. Within three days, Jennifer W.M. revived. She breathed easily. Her hands were steady (warm, too), her eyes sparkled romantically, and she walked and acted with the vitality of a young woman. She felt she had been "restored to life" again with the help of this cell-feeding "C + Iron Tonic."

BALLOON BREATHING BUILDS STRONGER BLOOD CELLS

You Will Need: A simple balloon. Get the very thick kind that calls for a lot of strenuous blowing.

How to Do It: Breathe in through your nose and fill up your lungs. Then blow out air into the balloon until it is filled. Relax as you let the air out of the balloon, then repeat. Plan to balloon breathe for a full ten minutes each day. Gradually, increase the time to 15 minutes.

Cellular Benefits: The deep inhalation floods your 750 million air sacs (or cells) with oxygen. The oxygen travels through the cells to get into your bloodstream. Your red and white blood cells now absorb the oxygen content of the air, and use it for self-regeneration. These oxygenated blood cells now work swiftly (the air revived and energized them) to cleanse away the stagnant clumps throughout your bloodstream. Within moments, the blood washing process takes place, thanks to this "fun" way of oxygenating your circulatory system.

Inhalation Programs Create New Will to Live

Walking with a stooped posture, looking bleary-eyed, Will D.E. appeared to be aging at an alarming rate. A consulting engineer, he found it difficult to concentrate on blueprints, and was confused with the simplest of mechanical terms. His professional status was jeopardized by his declining health. He felt so drained, that at times he said he just had no desire to continue on. It was as if he had lost the will to live.

A physiotherapist suggested he revive his bloodstream with a simple inhalation program. This would introduce nourishing oxygen into his air-starved blood cells. Within moments, the alerted cells would perform the needed debris-sweeping and waste-washing functions. Will D.E., desperate, followed the inhalation program. He did the deep breathing, and tried the balloon program. Almost at once, he felt himself revive. His posture became better; his face perked up; he looked younger. In three days on this cellular oxygenation program, he bounced back with renewed vigor. Now he had a new will to live. His cleansed bloodstream made him sparkle with the joy of life. All this through easy (and free) inhalation!

"TRIPLE-ACTION BLOOD-WASHING POTION"

Just three ingredients, in this unique combination, can revitalize your bloodstream and give you sparkling clean internal rivers. To prepare and enjoy, here are the easy instructions.

In a glass of grapefruit juice, add one tablespoon of desiccated liver, plus one teaspoon of brewer's yeast. Stir vigorously or blenderize for just 20 seconds. Drink it about an hour before your main meal.

Benefits: The Vitamin C of the juice combines with the iron and Vitamin B12 of the liver, as well as the B-complex of the brewer's yeast, to regenerate and reactivate your red blood corpuscles. They work together to supply your body with important cleansing oxygen to scrub your bloodstream clean. They also enhance your power of vesicular breathing, which means that your blood vessels are also washed, thus getting rid of more sediment.

In potion form, the liquefied ingredients are assimilated rapidly to provide you with this cleansing reaction. The three ingredients create a triple-action blood washing that will help you feel warm, alive and throbbing with the vitality of a young person . . . at any age.

You may not be able to see your bloodstream, but you can feel the rewards of having it washed when you experience that "great to be alive" feeling that comes with this cleansing. With the help of nutrition, water, inhalation, you can revitalize your bloodstream and your entire body.

BASIC POINTS

1. Garlic is a concentrated source of two blood cleansers that make it a powerful washing food.
2. Marcia J.H. corrected body chills by cleaning her blood with garlic.
3. Wash and "iron" your bloodstream with the simple, two-part, outlined program, in the privacy of your own home, in less than 30 minutes for speedy results.
4. For top-notch washing, combine Vitamin C plus iron in the life restoring "C + Iron Tonic." It made Jennifer W.M. become alive again.
5. Oxygenate your tired blood cells and improve their cleansing power in minutes. Try the fun-filled balloon breathing program, too. Both of these inhalation programs gave Will D.E. a new "will to live."
6. Revitalize and cleanse your rivers of life with the "Triple-Action Blood-Washing Potion."

CHAPTER **13**

Cleanse Your Arteries and Enjoy
a "Second Youth"

Clean debris away from your arteries and you immediately experience the joy of a "second youth" from head to toe. Your arteries are elastic tubes. Their task is to carry oxygen-reinforced fresh blood from your heart to all parts of your body. To fulfill this rejuvenating-nourishing obligation, they must be kept as free from sediment as possible. Only then are they able to maintain this vital total body nourishment for the look and feel of youthful health. But errors in daily living may cause wastes to accumulate in your body's "pipelines" and this poses a risk to your basic health.

WASTE OVERLOAD = CLOGGED ARTERIES

Wastes from the incompletely metabolized byproducts of undesirable foods may start to accumulate on the insides of the artery walls. These wastes eventually form into fatty deposits. These deposits become gradually thicker and thicker as they attract even more deposits. If this waste overload continues, the inside walls of your arteries become so clogged that the blood cannot move along at a normal rate. As the space inside the arteries grows smaller, more pressure is exerted on the blood, giving rise to the condition known as high blood pressure or hypertension.

Danger Symptoms Clogged arteries with choked-up blood deposits create symptoms such as cramps or tingling, sharp aches or pains when you want to move your arms or legs. Mental disorders such as memory lapses and fuzzy thinking are caused when these wastes accumulate on the arteries leading to your brain. Your vital organs (heart, kidneys, liver) also receive unpleasant reactions when the wastes gather on arteries leading to these areas. Since these organs are not being nourished with enough blood because of waste-choked arteries, they become ill, and so does the rest of you.

Prolonged Sediment Accumulation Threatens Life   As more and more sediment collects on the walls of your arteries, they pose the risk of projecting right into your bloodstream, forming a life-threatening blockage. Or, these wastes may break off in chunks and float around in your blood. If the wastes float toward a smaller blood vessel, they become lodged between the walls. This can cause a serious stroke that may be crippling or fatal! So do realize that prolonged sediment accumulation on and within your arteries can present the most dangerous of threats to your life.

ARTERIOSCLEROSIS—EXCESS SLUDGE ACCUMULATION

In this condition, there is the slow and steady pileup of wastes. The arteries become narrow and hard. They lose their flexibility. There is a buildup of plaques in the arterial walls, which may cause an occlusion (literally, a cutting off) of blood flow. This is the forerunner of a crippling form of cardiovascular disease such as coronary heart trouble.

Neglect Worsens Problem   A typical plaque may break apart. It then spews out dead wastes and sludge into the artery. This upsets the blood flow and causes platelets to collect at the site of the breakage. These stick to each other and to the wall to fill the channel. Parts of half-formed thrombi (wastes) may break loose from the wall and lodge in a plaque-narrowed part of the artery.

The arterial wall, weakened by formation of dense plaques, may bulge and bleed (to form an aneurysm or a ballooning-out of the wall of a vein) or burst completely. Spasms, a temporary closing of the blood vessels, may occur. Your very life now faces a serious threat as the waste sludge accumulates until it can actually choke off your blood circulation. So you can readily appreciate the importance of having clean arteries—they are the lifeline of health.

CAN FOOD MAKE YOU FEEL YOUNG FOREVER?[1]

Certain foods have the ability to keep your arteries clean and help you feel young forever. This is the discovery made by Julian Whitaker, M.D., director of the California (San Clemente) Health Treatment Center. He has found that a high-carbohydrate, low-fat food program is able to promote cleansing and heal many so-called "incurable" ailments and also give you many years of feeling young and active.

Basic Program: "My patients are put on a supervised program in which complex carbohydrates make up 80% of their calorie intake. The balance is made up of low-fat, low-cholesterol and low-protein foods." *Note:* Complex carbohydrates are found in whole grain breads and cereals, corn, and potatoes, as well as fresh fruits and vegetables.

Improves Heart Health   Dr. Whitaker labels fat as a villain in heart health and a cause of waste overload. "When large amounts of fat are eaten, the red blood cells stick together and stack up. This is called 'rouleaux formation' which limits the flow of blood cells through the capillaries. It creates 'sludging' with a 30% reduction of oxygen supply to the heart." The doctor suggests a low-fat intake as a means of boosting better oxygen supply so the heart can be nourished. This will create a "forever young" feeling of basic health.

Arteriosclerosis and Cholesterol   "Clogged arteries may be reversed eventually by reducing fat intake in your diet. Cholesterol levels can be brought down 30 to 40% so that your risk of heart disease may be reduced and eliminated." *Simple Plan:* Dr. Whitaker accomplishes this arterial cleansing by putting his patients on a high whole grain and natural carbohydrate food program, but with very low amounts of fats.

Be Careful About Fat   Dr. Whitaker says, "My studies show that if you drink just one glass of cream—or a beverage or food containing this amount of cream—your oxygen supply drops so much that

---

[1] *Natural Health Bulletin*, Delta Group, 1101D State Road, Princeton, N.J. 08540, January 1980. Available by subscription.

you may run the risk of an angina attack! If you eat a high-fat breakfast of ham, fried eggs and buttered toast, the same reaction may occur. In addition to your heart, all of your body tissues may become clogged. Your overall health declines." Dr. Whitaker urges you to reduce fat intake and thereby reduce waste intake to be rewarded with cleaner arteries and a healthier lifestyle.

Food Supplements Are Cleansing   Dr. Whitaker finds that some supplements spur an artery-cleansing reaction. He puts his patients on this supplement program:

Vitamin C. 1000 to 2000 milligrams with each meal, or a total of 3000 to 6000 milligrams daily.

Vitamin E. "A natural antioxidant," says Dr. Whitaker, "that boosts the use of cleansing oxygen, protects against certain cancers, and helps delay the aging process. Take 400 units daily in any form, although the dry preparations may be better."

Vitamin B-complex. From 10 to 20 milligrams of B1, B2, B6 and niacinamide daily.

Vitamin A. From 10,000 to 15,000 units daily.

Vitamin D. 400 units daily.

What About Minerals?   "Choose a mineral supplement that supplies zinc, chromium, and selenium along with other trace elements. We suggest you check with your physician, though, before starting any supplement program," advises the doctor.

RESULTS ARE CLEANSING

"At the beginning of a 12-day session at our center, blood tests are taken with most folks having cholesterol levels of 250 and over. The results at the end of the sessions are cleansing and remarkable. It's not unusual to see cholesterol levels drop from 250 to 150. This is all a result of the diet and the exercise program that is followed daily." Dr. Whitaker adds, "I gave up surgery because I feel diet and exercise are the ultimate ways to health. Our center is devoted entirely to this new life style to boost better and 'feel-young-forever' health."

Rewards: Says Dr. Whitaker, "With this diet program, most folks can say goodbye to many other low-oxygen symptoms such as fatigue, depression, confusion, lethargy and, in many cases, low sex drive." All this and much, much more in the way of refreshing young health is possible when you follow the program and cleanse your arteries and entire body, too.

HOW SIMPLE EXERCISES CAUSE ARTERY SCRUBBING IN DAYS

Keep yourself physically active, do mild exercises, and you can begin an artery-scrubbing reaction within a matter of days. The reason these programs work is because simple body movements cause an oxygenation of your body and this protects against an overloading of toxemia.

Oxygen Lack = Artery Clogging   Biologically speaking, an oxygen lack weakens the lining of the artery, making it more susceptible to clogging. Whenever there is an increased amount of sediment in the blood, it becomes incorporated into the wall of the red blood cell, thickening it. This thick wall makes it difficult to move oxygen from the red blood cells into the tissues. In other words, sediment makes the skin of the red blood cell "tough" and the cleansing oxygen cannot pass through it to the lining of the artery.

Problem: Red blood cells are the major carriers of oxygen to body tissues. If they cannot release this oxygen, the lining of the arteries becomes more vulnerable to sludge accumulation.

Solution: Increase the oxygen content of your blood and its oxygen-carrying ability through the use of regular exercise. This body movement will also boost the use of oxygen in your tissues which then releases more energy.

How Exercise Creates Oxygenated Cleansing   When you perform simple body motions, you boost the oxygen-carrying capacity of your bloodstream instantly. This automatically helps dissolve and wash out the sludge that accumulates in and on your arteries. The same oxygen will not only wash out wastes from your arteries, but help cleanse those in your bloodstream. Your red blood cells become healthier. Their own membranes now become healthfully thin and are able to pass oxygen more speedily. By providing a suitable supply of oxygen to the lining of your arteries, they are able to become cleansed and more resilient. You will have sparkling clean lifelines of health all because of exercise-prompted oxygen.

WHY TRIGLYCERIDE CONTROL IS IMPORTANT TO ARTERIAL YOUTHFULNESS

Lower your triglyceride levels and your arteries will be spared their sludge-like accumulations. Triglycerides are little-known blood fats that are transported through your vascular system, more so than the familiar cholesterol. Daily, some 70 to 150 grams of these waste-forming substances enter your body because you have consumed food from two taboo groups: (1) refined carbohydrates such as sugars and starches and (2) hard animal-source fats. This creates *hypertriglyceridemia* (elevated level of triglycerides in your blood) and the clogging of your arteries which is a life-threatening situation.

Simple Adjustment Solves Problem   Avoid any foods or beverages that contain refined carbohydrates. Read labels of packaged items. These are the waste-forming sugars and starches that make up the triglycerides and should be eliminated from your diet. *Tip:* You can enjoy carbohydrates but they should be of the complex variety such as whole grain breads and cereals and fresh fruits and vegetables—nothing processed. That's all there is to it!

Control Animal Fat Intake   These do create waste-forming triglycerides so just switch to vegetable fats. That is, liquid oils and products made from them. Meat is permissible in reasonable amounts but be sure to trim off all visible fat before cooking and then again before eating. Discover the joys of low-fat chicken, poultry and fish. High in polyunsaturates, vegetable oils wash away the artery-clogging triglycerides and help keep your arteries young. It's a simple change but it adds up to a lifetime of youthful health!

Lowers Dangerous Triglycerides in Seven Days

Constant trembling, nervous upset, fuzzy memory threatened the auditing position of Ronald I.B. He tired easily, even when sitting all day. He could scarcely keep his eyes open by midday.

Slightly overweight, he also looked haggard. He looked much more than his 50 years. A hematologist (blood specialist) diagnosed his problem as very high triglycerides. His arteries were being "choked to death!" Ronald I.B. was put on a simple two-step program: NO refined carbohydrate foods; NO animal fats. Within four days, he had a firm grip, was even tempered, and enjoyed a good memory. In seven days, he was alert, slimmed down, and presented the impression of a man looking younger than his formerly "old" 50 years. His triglyceride levels had dropped. His arteries were cleansed. Life was now so very wonderful.

THE CLEANSING POWER OF GARLIC

Ordinary garlic, whether chewed raw or used in cooking, creates a powerful cleansing action within your system. Garlic has a dilating effect on your blood vessels, scours away wastes, and helps to stabilize your pressure.

In particular, it is the *allicin* (the active sulfur-containing ingredient in garlic) that brings down the lipid (fat) levels in your bloodstream as well as in your vital organs. This helps break down the fatty clumps in your liver and other vital organs, and then releases them so that you have cleaner arteries.

Suggestion: Chew several garlic cloves daily. Remember to use parsley or even a cinnamon stick afterward to avoid becoming a social outcast. Use garlic as a salt substitute flavoring for most cooked foods (no odor when garlic is cooked). You can actually enjoy this way to cleaner arteries.

THE QUICK WAY TO CORRECT "METABOLIC SLUGGISHNESS" AND "SMOGGY OXYGEN"

These two problems are the forerunners to plaque or waste buildup. A weak metabolism and a waste-filled oxygen supply give toxemia a chance to accumulate. Since a more vigorous metabolism and strong oxygen availability help dislodge the wastes, it is important to find a way to create this situation. Otherwise, the situation in your body is similar to that of a stagnant pool. It becomes a cesspool of debris and is toxic to anyone who comes in contact with the putrid blockage. But there is a simple and very quick way to create an internal whirlpool that will actually dislodge and then wash out accumulated wastes. Here it is.

Wheat Germ Oil + Body Movements = Cleansing Metabolism   You know about the oxygenating power of ordinary wheat germ. But did you know this vegetable oil contains a dynamic cleansing ingredient called *octacosanol*? It is this magic substance that is able to whip up your metabolism and cleanse your "internal smog" to give you clean arteries. *Note:* When you take wheat germ oil and then do body movements or go for a fast walk, you promote a dynamic cleansing power within a matter of moments. It is this unique combination that can revitalize your entire body almost at once.

Magic of Octacosanol   This powerful cleansing ingredient found in wheat germ oil has the ability to transfer oxygen from the blood to your muscle tissues. It influences the release of oxygen in your muscles, too, and accelerates your metabolism. Octacosanol creates an internal "air conditioning" so that smoggy pollutants are blown away, so to speak. You are left with a refreshingly good feeling. It is similar to the sparkling sunshine after a sudden thunderstorm has ended. Everything is so fresh and pure and clean. So it is with your body, thanks to the magic of octacosanol—and it is found in ordinary wheat germ oil.

Basic Cleansing Program   Daily, just take from two to four tablespoons of wheat germ oil either as a salad dressing, or mixed with tomato juice. Then plan to go for a 30- to 60-minute walk. The combination of the octacosanol and the metabolic alertness caused by the physical activity is like treating your arteries to a complete housecleaning. Within moments, you'll look and feel healthfully alert. Your wastes will be evaporated and your arteries will be young again. So will you.

Overcomes Arteriosclerosis, Restores Youth

Told by her internist that she had dangerously high blood fat levels and thick porridge-like clumps of wastes that were choking her arteries, Helga DeH. was eager to correct this hazard. She followed her internist's diet guidelines calling for low- or no-animal fat foods. She also took the octacosanol-rich wheat germ oil and went for 60-minute walks twice a day. Within nine days, Helga

DeH. was diagnosed as having youthful arteries, cleansed of waste. She was the picture of health, too. She felt that her youthfulness was restored, thanks to this easy and speedy cleansing technique.

Clean Arteries Today—Youthful Life Tomorrow Protect your lifelines from sludge and you will enjoy an oxygenated and blood-nourished circulatory system. These artery cleansing programs work swiftly and effectively. Begin today and you will experience the joys of youth tomorrow.

IN A NUTSHELL

1. Control triglyceride levels and you will have cleaner arteries. Ronald I.B. followed a two-step program that reduced these levels and made him youthfully healthy again.

2. Garlic helps cleanse wastes and thereby control blood pressure.

3. Wheat germ oil (a prime source of cleansing octacosanol) and simple body movements, such as walking, exert a dynamic cleansing action in minutes. This easy program helped Helga DeH. overcome arteriosclerosis and enjoy restored youth.

14

How Body Motions Wash Away Stubborn Aches and Pains

Wash away accumulated debris clinging to your cells and tissues and you will be able to help ease and erase stubborn aches and pains. Muscle tissues often become cluttered with metabolic wastes that cause irritation erupting in the form of backaches, leg cramps, neck pains and a general feeling of being achy. The cause may be traced to an inactive lifestyle. It is similar to rust on an item not much in use. The rust clings to the item, making it difficult to handle if it has to be used. Only when the rust is washed away, can the item be used with more flexibility. So it is with your cells, your vital organs, your muscular system. You need to keep them active so that any "rust" (metabolic wastes) that does accumulate, can be shaken loose and washed out of your body.

REGULAR BODY MOTIONS PROTECT AGAINST RECURRING ACHES

When you follow some simple body motions or exercise programs, you dislodge stubborn wastes and cleanse the related systems and organs so there is less impingement of your movements. Body motions help you free yourself from these ache-causing wastes. Some benefits of these easy-to-do body motions are:

* You'll cleanse your blood circulation. This helps your vital organs and muscles work together more efficiently, without any sediment-causing pains.

* Exercise helps wash away dirt from your nerve cells. You will then be able to handle routine stresses more readily.

* Simple exercises dislodge toxic wastes from your bones, ligaments, and tendons. You will have clean organs that can function without grating pain.

* With a cleansed system, your vital organs respond more smoothly. Body motions or exercises stimulate your cleansed lungs to absorb more oxygen. Your blood is improved by an increase in hemoglobin. This leads to an additional supply of oxygen to your muscles. Cleansed, they are able to contract and expand without painful reactions.

* There are bonus benefits as you develop an improved self-conception and body image. You enjoy more vitality, increased self-confidence and the joy of living.

These are a few of the rewards you experience when simple body motions uproot and shake loose the stubborn "body rust" that causes distressing aches and pains.

EASY BODY MOTIONS CLEANSE AWAY BURSITIS TOXEMIA

Bursitis is traced to the accumulation of calcium-like wastes that have accumulated in certain pockets of your body. A *bursa* is a sac situated between two structures, such as between skin and bone, between bone and tendons, and so on. In many situations, incompletely metabolized calcium or accumulated wastes tend to gather in the bursa, giving rise to pain.

While you have these bursa pockets in your elbows, your hips, and your knees, the most common area of distress is around your shoulder. In most cases, these calcium wastes accumulate in one of the tendons that elevates your arm when you need to put on your coat, reach in a back pocket or brush your hair. There is a sharp pain, which is caused by the grating irritation of these refuse wastes that block the free movement of your arms. To correct this, it is helpful to use some simple body motions. These cleanse away bursitis toxemia and give you cleansed tendons, the key to youthful flexibility.

Horizontal Arm Circles

Position: Stand erect, arms extended sideward at shoulder height, palms up.

Body Motion: Make small circles backward with hand and arms. Reverse, turn palms down and do small circles forward. Repeat 15 to 20 times.

Shrug Away Bursitis Pain

Position: Stand erect, hands at sides.

Body Motion: Gently rotate your shoulders up, back, down and around. Repeat 10 to 15 times.

Arm Swing and Flex

Position: Stand erect, arms at sides, hands upward at chest level.

Body Motion: Swing both arms together forward and back. On the forward swing, flex both elbows, drawing your fists toward your shoulders. *Note:* Inhale while your arms swing forward and back. Exhale vigorously as you bring them down again. Repeat 15 times.

Book Holding for Shoulder Freedom

Position: Stand erect, arms extended overhead. Hold a book in each hand.

Body Motion: (1) Bend arms at elbows, slowly lowering your book-holding hands. (2) Keep your elbows as high as possible, close to your head. (3) Extend arms slowly as you return to starting position. Repeat 3 sets up to 10 times.

Cleanses, Refreshes, Restores Flexibility These easy body motions are directed at cleansing away the crystal-like wastes that are inhibiting the full range of motion for your shoulders. You will feel refreshed as the dislodged toxic wastes are broken up and eliminated from your body. With restored flexibility, you can say goodbye to waste-caused bursitis.

Eight Years of Bursitis Conquered in Eight Days

Doing ordinary household chores became agony for Adele Y.C. as the years rolled on. Her shoulder pains were so intense, she would scream and then sob when she had to make an unexpected upper body movement. She thought she would become an invalid because of her bursitis. A physiotherapist suggested she loosen up the clogging deposits and cast them out of her bursa pockets. This would get to the cause of her problem. Adele Y.C. followed the easy body motions as described above. Amazed, her flexibility was restored within a few days. At the end of eight days she was as vigorous as a youngster. She did, indeed, conquer her agonizing bursitis problem of eight years in just eight days.

EASY LEG-ERCISES TO MELT AWAY
TOXEMIA-CAUSED CRAMPS

Those stiff legs that make you feel helpless are in need of washing. Not externally, but internally. That is, the accumulation of wastes in your legs often become locked in joints, ligaments, tendons, cells, and even in the bloodstream. Here, they become glue-like in their stubbornness as they restrict free movement of your legs. You know that it is toxemia when you experience a sharp, stabbing sensation while trying to bend your knees. Often, in the middle of the night, you experience severe cramps. And the most obvious symptom is chronic tiredness and leg weakness after walking just a short distance. You need to uproot and cast out the accumulated toxic wastes. Here is a set of fun-to-do body movements. They are aimed at unlocking debris from your hips right down to your toes. Within moments, you will feel the heaviness lifted and a more youthful flexibility in your legs. When you wash out the debris, you restore strength and comfort to your legs.

Quick Leg Revitalization Movement
Position: Stand on one foot, holding onto something for balance. Keep your back straight.
Body Motion: Using your free hand, pull your knee toward your chest. Don't strain. Get an easy stretch. Gradually, increase the action from 10 to 30 seconds. Repeat three times.

Lower Leg Rejuvenation
Position: Put the ball of your foot on the edge of a curb or stair, with the remaining part of your foot hanging down over the edge.
Body Motion: Lower heel down below level of curb where the ball of your foot is resting. Go slowly, working on balance. You may need to hold onto something for balance. Keep leg on which your Achilles tendon and ankle are being stretched as straight as

possible. Stretch is the easy phase. Be relaxed before increasing the stretch. Work on feeling a good stretch. Slowly does it. Repeat up to 5 times.

Easy Knee Bend

Position: Stand erect, hands on hips, feet comfortably spaced.

Body Motion: Bend knees to 45°, keeping your heels on the floor. Return to starting position. Do it again. Repeat 10 to 15 and gradually 20 times.

Calf Raise

Position: Stand erect, hands on hips, feet spread 6 to 12 inches apart.

Body Motion: Raise your body up on your toes, lifting your heels. Return to starting position. Keep breathing deeply. Repeat up to 5 sets. This is a simple, yet remarkably exhilarating exercise that dislodges and eliminates wastes promptly, restoring youthful flexibility and freedom from pain to your lower limbs.

Frees Legs of Lifetime Pain in Six Days

Nearly crippled by agonizing leg pains, Hugo O'N. had such stiffness in his legs that he was either confined to a chair or would soon face the gloomy prospect of having to use a wheelchair. Standing or walking for a short distance brought such cramps, he had to sit down and gasp for breath. Fearing inevitable crippling, he sought help from a newly established holistic health practitioner, one who treated the entire body instead of just the symptoms. The physician tested Hugo O'N. and diagnosed his problem as sludge deposits that were glued together in his lower cell-tissue extremities, causing serious blockages. He prescribed the set of leg-ercises. Hugo O'N. followed them. Immediately, he felt the "shackles" removed from his legs. In just six days, he was totally free of the crippling pains. To celebrate, he entered a jogging marathon and finished second! Just 20 to 30 minutes of leg-ercises daily washed away the toxemic blockages and transformed him from an invalid to a champion!

CASTING OUT "PHANTOM ACHES"

An ache that appears suddenly, then just as suddenly is gone, only to appear elsewhere in your body is a much-disliked and feared phantom ache.

Basic Cause: Your blood system is overburdened with accumulated toxic wastes. As blood flows throughout your body, its sediment spills over and becomes fixed on your muscles, tendons, cells, tissues, bones. These toxic wastes often clump together, sometimes for a brief time only. A sudden ache is the reaction. Soon, the clump dissolves only to find another gathering site. This is the location of a repeat ache. This "phantom" situation calls for simple body motions to help promote better elimination of wastes.

Carry out as many of the following motions each day as it is comfortable to do. They are aimed at breaking up toxic clumps and speeding their elimination.

Seated Toe Touch. With toes pointed, as you sit on a carpeted floor, slowly slide hands down legs until you feel the stretch. Hold position and bob lightly to increase stretch. Grasp ankles and slowly pull until your head approaches your legs. Relax. Draw your toes back. Slowly attempt to touch toes. Repeat 5 times.

Knee Pull. Pull leg to chest as you sit on a carpeted floor, and hold for a count of 5. Repeat with opposite leg (8 to 10 times for each leg).

Toe Pull. Seated on the carpeted floor, pull on your toes while pressing legs down with your elbows.

Wall Stretch. Stand 3 feet from wall, with feet slightly apart. Put both hands on wall. With heels on ground, lean forward slowly and feel stretch in calves. Hold position for 15 to 20 seconds. Repeat several times.

Standing Toe Touch. Stand with legs straight and *slowly* bend over and reach for your toes as far as is comfortably possible. Hold for count of 5—bob lightly. Straighten up. Repeat several times.

Side Bender. Extend one arm overhead, other on hip. Slowly bend to side; bob gently to loosen up and shake debris out of pockets. Repeat 5 times for each side.

Jumping Jack. Stand with arms at side. On count 1, jump and spread feet apart and simultaneously swing arms over head. On count 2, return to starting position. Use a rhythmic, moderate cadence. Repeat 15 to 25 times.

30 Minutes Daily Preferably either after breakfast or about one hour before your evening meal, this set of exercises will do much to dislodge wastes and ease their elimination. Once removed, your body is free of debris-causing "phantom aches."

WASHING (THE INSIDES) OF YOUR FEET FOR FREEDOM FROM ACHES

You wash the outsides of your feet. Good. Now you need to wash the insides. That is, with the use of simple exercises, you can increase the circulation flowing to your feet and boost a cleansing reaction that will do away with recurring aches. Remember, your feet are furthest from your heart, so they are usually the first to become sluggish because of waste pileup. With simple foot exercises, you can wash away the accumulated debris and help yourself feel much better.

Why Exercises Are Helpful Sluggish circulation delays cellular cleansing and replacement. Products such as lactic acid and other debris become lodged in your arteries and venous system, blocking blood from returning to your heart. This can cause painful reactions. The following exercises help your muscles pump blood back to your heart. They also open your venous valves to promote a freer exchange of oxygen and waste, causing a subsequent internal washing. Your feet are stronger and you feel glad all over.

1. Sit, relaxed, with bare feet on your carpeted floor or on a towel. Try to pick up a pencil with your toes. *Benefit:* Washes tendons on top of your foot.

2. Sit in a relaxed position. Cross one leg over the other. Bend your top foot down and then up. Rotate your foot in one direction, then another. Do this up to 15 times for each foot. *Benefit:* Washes wastes from ankle joints to relieve stiffness.

3. Stand on bare feet. Rise up on your toes, and then back down again. Repeat 10 times. *Benefit:* Cleanses debris from your ankles and arches.

4. Stand. Roll your feet outward up to 15 times until your weight rests comfortably on the outer borders of your feet. *Benefit:* Washes away debris from your inner arches to relieve strain.

5. Stand with feet together. Bend toes up as far as you can up

to 10 times. *Benefit:* Cleanses away toxic wastes from the muscles of your toes.

6. Stand. Keep both knees stiff as you cross your legs (as a scissors) with feet flat on the floor and slightly apart. Distribute your body weight evenly between both feet. Hold this position for a count of 30. Reverse. *Benefit:* Helps cleanse away impediments from the muscles controlling foot and leg balance.

7. Sit on a carpeted floor with both legs extended straight ahead. Bend your feet upward as far as is comfortably possible. *Benefit:* Washes cells of the calf and heel muscles.

8. Sit on a carpeted floor with both legs extended straight ahead. Turn the soles of your feet closely together (as if clapping your soles together). *Benefit:* Cleanses debris from arches and tones up calf muscles through tendon-ligament washing.

9. Lean against a wall. Put your weight on your arms. Now, kick yourself gently in the upper thigh. Easy does it. Do this with each foot. *Benefit:* Helps dislodge wastes in your thigh muscles and promote greater flexibility.

10. Lie flat on carpeted floor or on a bed. Bend your knee. (That grating noise is a dislodging of nitrogenous wastes.) Grasp your leg with both hands. Gently pull your knee back towards your body.

30 Minutes Daily   That's all you need to promote washing of the insides of your feet. You will be able to boost important metabolic reactions to exhilarate your lower limbs and the rest of your body.

PAIN-FREE HIGHLIGHTS

1. Adele Y.C. overcame eight years of bursitis by performing easy body motions for only eight days.
2. Melt away toxemia-caused cramps with easy leg-ercises. Hugo O'N. freed his legs of lifetime pain in just six days with this simple at-home program.
3. Cast out "phantom aches" with easy waste-washing body motions.
4. Free your feet from aches with "inside washing" exercises. Just 30 minutes daily gives you total body fitness.

CHAPTER **15**

How to De-Age Your Cells and Make Your Body Brand New Again

Every part of your body is made of cells. The cleaner your cells, the younger your body. Since your trillions of cells are involved with your vital functions, you can understand the importance of using home programs for inner washing. With sparklingly fresh cells, you are rewarded with an equally sparkling and youthfully fresh body.

CLEAN CELLS = TOTAL REJUVENATION

You have cells whose chief task is to take in valuable oxygen. You have cells whose main function is to receive and dispatch stimuli. You have cells which work to help you contract or expand your muscles. You have cells which release fluids, and cells which transport nutrients from one part of your body to another. Some cells carry iron in hemoglobin to nourish your bloodstream. In order to perform these tasks, your cells need to be clean of accumulated wastes. Then they will be able to fulfill their obligations in keeping your body healthy, repairing your vital organs, and building up immunity to illness, and making you look and feel youthfully alert.

Cells Influence Health Levels   Each cell has its own health job to perform. One cannot be substituted for another. One group of cells will ingest oxygen and food; another group will release wastes. It is important to have clean cells since they determine your level of health.

Looking at Your Cells   To know how to keep your cells clean, here are some basics about this smallest unit of your body that is capable of independent life. A cell is a tiny jelly-like blob. It consists of *cytoplasm*, a protein solution, in a fine but strong container called the *membrane*. Most cells have a dense kernel, the *nucleus*, which influences the activity of the rest of the unit. A cell contains a set of *organelles*, visible only with an electron microscope. These are tiny structures which have enclosing membranes, hardly more than a molecule thick.

Foundation of Your Health   Among the organelles found deep within your cells are mitochondria. This is the target zone or the bullseye of your health. It is in your mitochondria that nutrient combustion takes place to provide energy and vitality for your cell's activities. This means, that if your mitochondria structures are sparklingly clean and are able to create this nutrient metabolism, your cells can become super-invigorated and be able to perform at top efficiency levels. Your reward is a look and feel of complete youthful vitality. So you can readily appreciate the importance of having clean cells so you have healthy mitochondria structures. Your entire body will react with energy and stamina.

THE VITAMIN THAT RESTORES "YOUNG POWER" TO YOUR CELLS

Vitamin C is unique in being able to provide your organelles with a supercharge of energy so that you are filled with "young power" from head to toe.

Provides Energy, De-Aging, Cellular Rejuvenation   When you nourish your cells with Vitamin C through foods and supplements, a dynamic reaction occurs almost at once. The Vitamin C prompts your mitochondria structures to start absorbing oxygen. The vitamin speedily urges your cells to burn oxygen so that wastes can be evaporated. Moments later, the Vitamin C promotes cellular rejuvenation. That is, it takes out the aged cells and replaces them with new ones. Vitamin C also rejuvenates your *osteoblasts*, which are bone-forming cells. Vitamin C also works to bring about the repair of all the fibrous or tissue parts of your body.

Without Vitamin C, the activities of the osteoblasts and fibroblasts (tissue makers) are diminished, even halted. This could lead to the aging problem. So it is important to have Vitamin C available at all times in suitable quantities to help protect against cellular aging.

VITAMIN C REBUILDS "AGING" SKIN CELLS

When Vitamin C enters your bloodstream, it speedily works at the task of preparing *collagen*. This is an abundant protein needed to repair your body tissues. Fibrous, tough and pliant, collagen (its name is derived from the Greek word for glue) is needed to rebuild your cartilage, bone, tendons, ligaments, arterial walls, nerve sheaths, and vital organs. It depends upon Vitamin C for the materials required in this reconstruction. When Vitamin C initiates the making of collagen, your aging cells can then be repaired and regenerated. But even more important, Vitamin C acts to scour, cleanse and wash your mitochondria structures. This helps "de-age" your cells and rejuvenate your entire body.

How Vitamin C Rejuvenates the Skin   When assimilated by your digestive system, Vitamin C is oxygen-transported via your bloodstream to your cells. The vitamin speedily promotes the mitochondria cleansing; then it is used to perk up aged skin. Vitamin C is absorbed by your body's own cells and blood vessels. Soon, it becomes a living part of your skin tissue, but before this can be done, your cells need to be cleansed so that Vitamin C can be absorbed through the cell membrane and enter the nucleus. When this is accomplished, your skin undergoes a transformation. It becomes firm, smooth and young again. You can see that rebuilding and rejuvenating your skin is an "inside" job, thanks to Vitamin C.

Fresh Citrus Juices Wash-Rebuild Cells   A powerful concentration of Vitamin C is found in fresh citrus juices. Use oranges, grapefruits, tangerines, lemons, and limes. Freshly squeezed citrus juice is a prime source of enzymes, too. These are protein-like miracle workers that energize Vitamin C and prompt it to perform its washing-rebuilding of your cells. Therefore, a few glasses of fresh citrus juice daily will exert a powerful influence on your mitochondria and boost the manufacture of cell-healing collagen.

Wonder Youth Tonic Rebuilds Body in Three Days

Christopher T.R. began to develop one ailment after another. Blotches cropped up all over his body. Digestive upsets made him skip meals and become malnourished. His nerves were very sensitive and he would snap upon the slightest provocation. His vision was blurred; he caught one cold after another. He walked like an old man with a "hunched" look because of his rounded shoulders. He showed all the signs of aging rapidly, even though he was not out of his early 50s. A local cytologist (specialist in cellular rebuilding) diagnosed his problem, which was waste-laden cells that could not be nourished because of toxic blockages. A simple program was prescribed: three times daily, he was to have a glass of a "Wonder Youth Tonic." Almost at once, Christopher T.R. responded. His skin cleared and tightened and became bright again. His digestion was good; he was cheerful again; his eyesight sharpened. He went without any sniffles and had a firm posture. The "hump" eventually straightened. At the end of three days, he felt as if 20 years had been taken off his life. All this because of the powerful elements in the tonic.

"Wonder Youth Tonic" To prepare, just squeeze, blenderize, or extract the juice from any citrus fruit. Try a combination of fruits, such as equal amounts of oranges, grapefruits, tangerines with a squeeze of either lemon or lime juice. Add a half teaspoon of honey for added flavor. *Special Boost:* Crush a 1000 milligram tablet of Vitamin C (from any health store) into the tonic for super-power. Just drink one glass after breakfast, another after your noon meal, and a third one at the end of your evening meal.

Restores Tissue Integrity, Cleanses, Refreshes The enzymes in the raw juice will dispatch the highly concentrated Vitamin C via your bloodstream to your trillions of cells. Here, the vitamin works swiftly to rebuild your cytoplasm, membrane, mitochondria, osteoblasts, and fibroblasts. At the same time, enzymes plus C will scour away accumulated wastes that otherwise block nutrient regeneration. It is this double action of: (1) restoration, and

(2) cleansing, that will exert an overall refreshing regeneration of your entire body. This is the power of the "Wonder Youth Tonic," especially when fortified with a Vitamin C tablet for super-cleansing, super-regeneration.

More Sources of Cell-Cleansing Vitamin C   This cleansing-regenerating vitamin is found in the papaya, strawberries, cantaloupe, tomato, broccoli, green peppers, raw leafy greens, white and sweet potatoes.

Plan to have a fresh fruit or raw vegetable salad each day. You will be introducing a high concentration of the important cell-cleansing and cell-rejuvenating Vitamin C. This works around-the-clock in the de-aging process. You will need to cook the broccoli and potatoes, and some Vitamin C will be evaporated, but you should include these foods, too. They help establish a good foundation for cellular cleansing.

WHY ANIMAL FATS ARE HARMFUL TO YOUR CELLS

An excessive amount of animal fats can be cell-destroying. The problem here is that these hard fats leave thick sludge right on your mitochondria. Your cells are unable to receive enough oxygen to burn foodstuffs completely to energy-producing carbon dioxide and water. Your waste-covered cells become "choked" and cannot survive. This causes the aging process. The normal enzyme activity is also altered and cellular deterioration worsens.

Simple Change Reverses Aging Process   Limit your intake of animal foods. Instead of too much butter, use vegetable margarine and oils. Switch to low-fat dairy products. Avoid skins of meat and poultry. Cook with vegetable oils only. Change from meats to more fish. In so doing, you will spare your cells the waste-forming fats that block free oxygen transfer. You can then help reverse the cellular aging process and cleanse your mitochondria to open the way to youth restoration.

Says "No" to Hard Fats, Says "Yes" to Eternal Youth

Irked by being called the "old man" in his office, Martin Z. took a close look at himself. He ruefully (and silently) admitted he did look like an old man with his pale skin, double chin, blotchy eyes, and general malaise. He took his problems to an internist who also advocated orthomolecular (total body) healing with an emphasis on nutrition. An exam and blood test showed that Martin Z. had "cellular clogging" because of hard fatty wastes gluing his mitochondria together, like a clogged up sieve. It blocked free transport of oxygen and nutrients. Cellular destruction was the cause of his aging. The internist put him on a simple program of no animal fats at all. He could enjoy fish because it was a source of valuable polyunsaturates with low hard fats. He was told to switch to free-flowing oils and products made from them. Martin Z. followed this dietary change. In four days, he developed a firm, youthful skin with no more sag, no more blotchy appearance, no more letdown. He had such vitality, he was called "wonder man" instead of "old man." The easy change has corrected his cellular deterioration, cleansed his body, and given him the look and feel of eternal youth.

HOW FISH OILS DE-AGE YOUR CELLS AND ADD YEARS TO YOUR LIFE

The use of fish oils is important in cellular cleansing. They are a prime source of Vitamin D, also known as the "sunshine vitamin" and this is needed to promote cell scouring and nourishment.

Fish Oils Revitalize Lymphatic System A unique, but powerful reaction takes place when you make fish oils available to your digestive system.

The oils cooperate with your lymphatic system. Their free flow bathes all of your body cells with a fluid that consists of antibodies and white blood cells. Your lymphatic system controls the levels of wastes in your body. It offers three powerful scouring actions. All require the power of Vitamin D from fish oils to function. These include:

1. *Blood Protein Cleansing.* The lymphatic system cleanses protein and then deposits it into your blood. You need clean protein to have a clean bloodstream and it is Vitamin D-energized lymphatics that create this reaction.

2. *Cleanses in Between Cellular Spaces.* Energized by Vitamin D, lymphatics cleanse spaces between your cells and discharge wastes such as toxins, bacteria, cholesterol, viruses. *Note:* Your lymphatics cleanse the fluid that is used to bathe every cell in your body.

3. *Boosts Resistance to Viral Infections.* Remember, a virus is a

waste product or germ that causes infections. You need to resist viruses. A Vitamin D-energized lymphatic system will stimulate your white cells (called lymphocytes) to circulate and destroy foreign wastes such as bacteria, parasites and dangerous viruses.

Energize Your Lymphatic System for Total Cleansing Immunity   This waste-washing, virus-fighting system is composed of a series of gland-like stations throughout your body. Sometimes called lymph nodes or glands, they are bean-shaped substances found in your neck, armpits, behind your knees, around your pelvic region, close to your arteries, surrounding your heart. All are connected by a network of slender-walled channels, which crisscross your entire body, especially near your arteries and veins. Flowing through the system is the fluid which is aptly named, *lymph*. Colorless, it contains nutrients that help protect against the starvation of your cells and helps them from aging. But this lymphatic system can become waste-burdened and sluggish.

Wastes Block Free Flow of Cleansing Lymph   An accumulation of wastes will slow down the lymph flow. The condition is known as *lymphstasis*. You can compare it to a clogged kitchen sink drain. If you let the water run, the sink overflows and spills onto the floor.

The same situation happens inside your body during lymphstasis. Accumulating fluid fills up spaces between your cells and is unable to be carried off by the lymphatics. *Problem:* There is a subsequent pileup of fluid and pressure in the intercellular spaces. *Reactions:* Lymph channels in your lungs become so engorged with fluid wastes, they start to stiffen. So will the vital left heart ventricle, which dispatches oxygen-carrying blood throughout your body. This can cause congestive heart failure, caused by *edema* or fluid buildup.

So you realize that accumulated wastes and liquids cause lymphstasis or stagnation and swelling, and cause the risk of body breakdown. Wastes act as dangerous blockages.

HOW FISH OILS IMPROVE LYMPH FLOW

As rich concentrates of polyunsaturated fatty acids and powerful Vitamin D, fish oils will stimulate your lymphatic system. They energize the lymphocytes to release substances such as *macrophages* (waste-washers) which devour the wastes and speed their elimination. Vitamin D from the fish oils increases the numbers of waste-washing lymphocytes, accelerates the creation of antibodies (debris-cleansing gamma globulins), and manufactures a powerful cleanser known as *interferon*.

Interferon as Natural Cell Washer   Vitamin D stimulates the lymphocytes to release the powerful cell cleanser known as interferon. This dynamic virus-fighter scours your cells and works with the macrophages to wash away wastes. All this is possible with the availability of Vitamin D from fish oils.

Sunlight or Vitamin D Supplements   Sunlight is a not-too-reliable source of Vitamin D if you happen to live in a part of the country that is cloudy or polluted, blocking out "Old Sol." It has been shown also that sunlight in high doses can be damaging to your skin cells. A moderate amount of sunlight is helpful, but while this is safer, it is not as concentrated a source of Vitamin D as is required. Therefore, use fish liver oils as a supplement. Or, ask at your health food store about supplements to be used with your doctor's guidance.

Simple Way to Boost Lymphatic Cleansing Powers   Mix three tablespoons of any fish liver oil (available at health stores or pharmacies) in a glass of fresh vegetable juice. Stir vigorously or blenderize for 20 seconds. Drink one glass daily. The enzymes in the juice will dispatch the Vitamin D into your metabolic system within moments after swallowing. Your lymphatic system becomes super-energized and is able to release important scouring substances. With cleansed cells, you build your immunity to aging. In a short time, you can give yourself a brand-new body, thanks to brand-new cells.

Conquers Lifetime Disabilities in 12 Days

Years and years of crippling allergies, and an inability to resist respiratory sensitivities, so weakened Jennifer J. that she was often confined to a chair. If she had to exert herself, it made her gasp for breath and need to lie down. Unhappily, she resorted to a wheelchair for going great distances. Saddened by the prospect of becoming an invalid, she sought help from a nutrition therapist. Tests showed that she had a serious decline in adequate lymphocytes.

Clogged cells locked out the free transfer of important nutrients. Jennifer J. was put on a simple program: eliminate all hard animal fats and take from 4 to 6 tablespoons of fish liver oil daily. She also had to drink fresh juices daily, too. Results? Within six days, she could walk unaided. She could breathe deeply. Within ten days, Jennifer J. was as vigorous as a youngster. She discarded her wheelchair. She was getting ready to jog by the twelfth day, having conquered her lifetime disabilities through cellular cleansing with Vitamin D.

REBUILD LYMPHATIC SYSTEM, REGENERATE CELLS, REJUVENATE BODY

Vitamin D helps exhilarate your lymphatic system to release scouring agents that cleanse and then regenerate your cells. By boosting your virus-fighting and germ-destroying powers, Vitamin D keeps your cells clean and this is your key to a rejuvenated body.

Everything you see and cannot see consists of cells. They are the controlling forces of your health. Keep them clean and nourished, and they will keep you more than just healthy, but invigoratingly youthful. Remember—whatever is good for your cells is good for every part of you!

IN A CAPSULE

1. Clean up your cells and enjoy total rejuvenation with the sets of outlined programs.
2. De-age your cells with the cleansing power of Vitamin C.
3. The tasty "Wonder Youth Tonic" rebuilt Christopher T.R.'s body in three days.
4. Martin Z. firmed up his body and corrected aging with the use of a simple program that eliminated excessive hard animal fats.
5. Fish liver oils energize your cleansing lymphatic system to fight infections.
6. Jennifer J. overcame lifetime disabilities in 12 days through cellular cleansing by boosting her lymphatic system via fish liver oils.

16

The 10¢ Magic Food That Performs Total Cleansing Within Hours

Fiber (or roughage, as our grandparents called it) is a dynamic cleansing food that can give you the feeling of sparkling good health within a few hours. Basically, fiber is a nutrient that is *not* digested to absorbable substances. Because of this trait, it is useful in sweeping away debris and assisting in its removal. It is this cleansing power that makes fiber a magic food in terms of internal rejuvenation. It works speedily, effectively, and with little effort on your part. The total cleansing results are magical.

MEET THIS DYNAMIC CLEANSER

What Is Dietary Fiber?   This is a term that is given to the components of a food that are not fully broken down by the enzymes in your digestive tract. This fiber is not digested by your body; instead, after it is eaten, it creates a sweeping-cleansing action as it passes through your body and is eliminated.

What Are Fiber Sources?   Plants such as grains, nuts, seeds, fruits, vegetables are good sources of fiber. All contain various amounts of this dynamic cleanser. Meats, fish, poultry, and dairy products (all of animal origin) contain no fiber.

What Does Fiber Consist Of?   Fiber is composed of hemicelluloses, pectic substances, gums, mucilages, and cellulose. Found largely in the cell walls of the plant foods, these substances are nondigestible in the sense that they do not remain in your system. Instead they cause an internal sweeping action as they pass through on the way to elimination.

FIBER: HOW IT DIGESTS, CLEANSES, HEALS

This nutrient is also known as "bulk" or "roughage" although it is not really rough. It does have a sweeping action in your digestive-intestinal system and it also does provide needed bulk. When you eat this magic food, it enters your digestive system where it becomes absorbed with available liquid. (It's important to have a liquid when consuming fiber foods.)

Fiber has a water-holding capacity that makes it an effective cleanser. It passes through your intestinal canal somewhat like a sponge, correcting and cleansing metabolism in the cecum (pouch in which the intestine begins). Here it remains for a brief time until ready for elimination, at which time the wastes, toxic debris, and pollutants it has picked up along the way are passed out as well.

This internal cleansing is able to initiate effective healing, since infectious debris is also scrubbed away from your vital organs.

Cleanses, Improves Gastrointestinal Tract When you ingest fiber, you initiate an important two-step cleansing reaction:

1. Fiber will help prevent waste-forming constipation by speeding up the transit time of food through your intestinal region. This is a major move in protecting against internal toxemia.

2. Fiber also eases straining at the stool. This helps protect you against such ailments as diverticular disease of the colon, irritable bowel syndrome, hemorrhoids, varicose veins, appendicitis, deep vein thrombosis, and hiatus hernia. With the use of fiber, the cleansing away of these wastes takes place in a short space of time. This reduces pressure and straining and toxic infection, and the cleansed gastrointestinal tract is able to reward you with youthfully good health.

DECREASED TRANSIT TIME IS SECRET OF FIBER'S MAGIC

This unique ability to create bulk and decrease the transit time of wastes and debris from storage to elimination makes it a dynamic cleansing food. This is the secret of its magic power in creating internal cleansing.

Dynamic Cleansing Action Since fiber holds water, wastes produced by a high-fiber diet tend to be bulkier and softer. The stools pass more quickly and easily through the intestines. This, in turn, means less strain and pressure on your bowels and blood vessels.

As the wastes move quickly through the intestines, surrounding tissues are less likely to be exposed to toxins. This decreased transit time protects your internal organs from overexposure to toxic substances and it is this dynamic cleansing action that makes fiber unique in its healing powers.

Fiber Helps Balance Cholesterol Levels An unusual power of fiber is in its ability to *decrease* the reabsorption of bile salts. These are substances needed to digest and emulsify fats and oils which then become absorbed into the intestines. But if you reabsorb too many bile salts, you run the risk of cholesterol overload.

Fiber Solves Problem Fiber compounds "bind" the bile acids and thereby reduce or prevent the reabsorption of bile acid, derived from your body's cholesterol. Reaction? Your body is then "ordered" to draw on its cholesterol stores to synthesize more bile acid. This helps lower your blood (serum) cholesterol levels. Since excess cholesterol may be considered as waste, it is important to use fiber to sweep it out and maintain healthier levels.

Controls Cholesterol, Cleanses Bloodstream on Fiber Program

His dangerously high cholesterol readings prompted Nicholas U. to seek help from a nutritionist. He was told that he had excessive blood sludge that would require speedy cleansing along with a lowering of his cholesterol level, another form of excess waste. Nicholas U. was put on a low animal fat program. But more important was the fiber program. Daily, Nicholas U. was to enjoy a plate of fresh raw vegetables sprinkled with two tablespoons of whole grain bran (from any health store or supermarket). He would continue eating most of his favorite foods. Within six days, his cholesterol level dropped down to a more healthy level. Within nine days, not only did he have a good cholesterol reading, but tests from the nutritionist showed a sparkling clean bloodstream. The fiber had swept away cholesterol wastes and blood sediment. In just nine days, he was refreshingly clean and youthful again.

EVERYDAY FOOD SOURCES OF CLEANSING FIBER

The use of fresh, raw, and unprocessed foods is essential for the fortification of cleansing fiber.

Raw Versus Refined   The emphasis is on raw foods. Refined or processed foods have had so much of the roughage taken out that they offer minimal amounts of this essential cleansing food. The raw foods create the desirable bulkier stools, more rapid transit, and lower intro-colonic pressures than the refined variety.

Here is a thumbnail grouping of good dietary fiber foods:

1. *Whole Grains.* This group refers to breads or cereals or grains that contain the entire product; that is, the bran or outer layer, the endosperm or starchy middle layers, the germ or fatty inner portion of the grain kernel.

2. *Vegetables.* These should be raw, whenever possible. If cooked, do so just enough to make them edible. *Tip:* Those vegetables that are "chewy" or "crunchy" when raw or slightly cooked are very high in cleansing fiber.

3. *Tuberous Root Vegetables.* This group includes carrots, parsnips, white and sweet potatoes, turnips, kohlrabi. *Tip:* The skin is high in fiber so try to retain this. Even if you do peel the vegetables, however, they are still prime sources of cleansing fiber.

4. *Fruits, Vegetables with Tough Skins.* If they contain edible seeds, they are very high in fiber. This group includes all varieties of berries, and also tomatoes, squash, eggplant.

5. *Pod Vegetables and Legumes.* Select from various green beans, green peas, dried beans and peas, lentils, lima beans, and others of this category.

6. *Seeds and Nuts.* You can eat those already shelled or those you need to shell. To derive top-notch fiber benefits, be sure to chew seeds and nuts very thoroughly.

THE SINGLE MOST CONCENTRATED SOURCE
OF CLEANSING FIBER

In a word—*bran.* It is the outer husk of grains. It comes from wheat, corn, rye, oat, rice, and so forth. This outer husk (or bran) is

Fiber in Selected Foods

Here is the fiber content of one serving (3½ ounces) of some fruits, berries and vegetables, nuts and seeds. We list only those which have a fiber content of one gram or more.

Food	Grams of fiber	Food	Grams of fiber
Almonds	2.6	Loganberries	3.0
Apples (not pared)	1	Macadamia nuts	2.5
Apricots (dried, uncooked)	3.8	Mustard greens (cooked)	1.0
Artichokes	2.4	Okra	1.0
Avocados	1.6	Olives	1.3
Beans, baked	1.5	Parsnips (cooked)	2.0
Beans, lima	1.8	Peanuts (with skins)	2.4
Beans, snap	1.0	Pears (including skin)	1.4
Beechnuts	3.7	Peas, snow	1.2
Beet greens (cooked)	1.1	Peas, cooked	2.0
Blackberries	4.1	Pecans	2.3
Blueberries	1.5	Peppers, raw	1.8
Brazil nuts	3.1	Popcorn	2.2
Broccoli	1.5	Prunes	2.2
Brussels sprouts	1.6	Raspberries	5.1
Cabbage, red	1.0	Rice bran	11.5
Carrots	1.0	Rice polish	2.4
Cashew nuts	2.6	Safflower seed meal	7.4
Celery	1.0	Seaweeds, dulse	3.2
Coconut meat	4.0	Irish moss	1.8
Collard greens	1.2	kelp	6.8
Cowpeas	1.8	laver	3.5
Cranberries	1.4	Sesame seeds, whole	6.3
Cress, garden	1.1	hull removed	2.4
Dandelion greens	1.6	Soybeans, cooked	1.6
Dates	2.3	natto	3.2
Figs (dried)	5.6	miso	2.3
Filberts	3.0	Squash, winter	1.8
Gooseberries	1.9	Strawberries	1.3
Guavas	5.6	Sunflower seeds	3.8
Kale	1.1	Walnuts, black	1.7
Lambs quarters (cooked)	1.8	English	2.1
Lentils	1.2		

a rich concentration of valuable cleansing fiber, almost without comparison to other foods.

Pure bran passes down into your lower bowel, absorbs water, adds bulk and then creates the valuable scouring-cleansing action throughout this entire region.

Unique Reaction   The power of bran is without equal as it causes acceleration of waste removal so that there is a reduced risk of bacterial infection. Otherwise, loitering microbes can cause deterioration of the gastrointestinal cells and open the way to ailments. But bran propels and discharges these wastes so there is a reduced incidence of waste infestation.

How Much Fiber in Bran?   In just 3½ ounces, you have over 9 grams of fiber. Since one ounce equals 2 tablespoons, you can make a simple calculation. Just 7 tablespoons of bran will give you at least 9 grams of this valuable scouring food.

10¢ a Day Keeps Body Youthfully Clean   Keep a "bran shaker" on your table. Throughout the day, sprinkle it over your foods. Mix it with juice or soups, on salads; use it in bread. Try it in yogurt, flavored with a bit of honey and fresh fruit. Add it to stews, casseroles, most baked goods.

The low cost means that for about 10¢ a day, you can keep your body youthfully clean and healthy. And bran has a delicious nut-like taste that makes food seem extra-special. You can actually eat your way to super health. . . and on just 10¢ a day, with bran.

Enjoys Regularity, Digestive Healing, Body Rejuvenation

Troubled by colitis, inability to eat even simple foods, recurring stomach pains, Oliver E.K. sought help from his gastroenterologist. His problem was waste overload as well as irritating debris. This body pollution was actually "eating away" at his delicate cellular membranes and tissue walls. His physician put him on an easy high-fiber food program. He was to have about 5 to 7 tablespoons of wheat bran daily over salads, in juices, soups, and baked goods.

Immediately, Oliver E.K. felt relief. Not only did he experience cleansing regularity, but his pains ended, and he began to feel more alert in body and mind. Within six days, he felt totally rejuvenated, thanks to the scouring-cleansing power of simple bran. It added a new taste to foods, too.

"MORNING BRAN BOOSTER TONIC"

In a glass of fresh vegetable juice, add two tablespoons of nonprocessed whole grain bran. Add a squeeze of lemon or lime juice for a piquant flavor. Blenderize for just 20 seconds and drink slowly right after your breakfast.

Cleansing Rewards The pure bran fiber is propelled by enzymes in the juice to scour and cleanse your digestive system in the morning. Your cells become washed and are now able to be renewed through the collagen-forming action of Vitamin C from fruits you eat later on. You will experience an inner cleansing and cellular rejuvenation that will make you feel younger than young!

From Slow Start to Top Speed in Three Days

Morning errors at her supervisory job threatened Joan McC.'s position. Her thinking was fuzzy; her speech was slurred; her movements were clumsy. This "slow start" extended almost till noontime. An efficiency expert suggested she boost her metabolism and cleanse away the blockages responsible for her sluggishness. Boosting her intake of fiber foods would help. Also each morning, she prepared the previously described tonic. Doing so, Joan McC. felt a revitalization almost at once. Within three days she was alert in body and mind, and worked so swiftly, she was recommended for a promotion! The "Morning Bran Booster Tonic" scoured her internal organs, helped regenerate her cells and tissues, and rejuvenated her metabolism. She was reborn, thanks to this 10¢ per portion "magic food."

DISCOVER WHEAT GERM: CELL CLEANSER SUPREME

Wheat germ is the seed of the wheat, containing a rich concentration of vitamins, minerals, protein, and the cell-cleansing fiber. In 3½ ounces (7 tablespoons), you have close to 3 grams of potent fiber, along with other cell-repairing nutrients.

Double-Action Cleansing Power Wheat germ contains octacosanol, a highly potent ingredient which works with fiber to cleanse away cholesterol, decrease transit time for waste removal, oxygenate your system, and bring about cellular repair so that you enjoy more vigor, stamina, and endurance. Octacosanol joins with fiber to scour your tissues, and then initiates the transfer of oxygen from your blood to those cleansed cells. This gives you the feeling of supreme health, all from the simple wheat germ.

Plan to use wheat germ daily to give yourself the important fiber to repair your cleansed cells and make you brand new again.

HOW TO USE BRAN AND WHEAT GERM FOR DAILY CELL CLEANSING

Here is a variety of ways to boost fiber intake with the use of both bran and wheat germ. Again, the cost is about 10¢ a day. The convenience is obvious, and the results will be felt right away.

- Prepare a mixture of wheat germ and bran in skim milk; add sesame seeds and sun-dried raisins.
- Stir one tablespoon of bran into your scrambled or poached eggs.
- Boost fiber power by adding bran and/or wheat germ to your pancake or waffle batter.
- Mix bran and wheat germ with seeds in a cup of plain yogurt.
- Use bran instead of croutons as part of a salad.
- Add to baked meat or fish or vegetable loaves.
- Use as a substitute whenever a recipe calls for cracker or bread crumbs.
- Add to a portion of cottage cheese and sliced fresh vegetables.
- When baking bread products or even cakes, include wheat germ and bran. For each cup of flour, use up to two tablespoons of either. That is, put these two tablespoons in your measuring cup, then add your whole grain flour. The taste will be superb, and the cleansing power extra-special, too.

When you think of fiber, just think of bran and wheat germ as the super-magic foods that can help perform total cleansing of your body within a matter of hours. Include the other listed fiber foods and you'll be rewarded with a brand new body. For less than 10¢ a day, you can receive good health. Fiber is your pot of gold at the end of the rainbow of youth.

IN A NUTSHELL

1. Meet fiber, a powerful cell cleanser and waste remover.
2. Nicholas U. was able to control his cholesterol level and

cleanse his bloodstream in just nine days on a simple fiber program.

3. Just 10¢ a day buys you enough powerful bran for total cleansing. It corrected Oliver E.K.'s problems of irregularity and digestive distress in a few days.

4. The "Morning Bran Booster Tonic" revitalized Joan McC. within three days so that she overcame her slowness and became an efficient worker.

5. Wheat germ is a tasty nugget of packaged health that is brimming with fiber. Use it daily and receive around-the-clock cellular cleansing and rejuvenation.

CHAPTER 17

The Raw Juice Way to Super Cleansing and Healthy Youth . . . at Any Age

Fresh fruit and vegetable juices are powerhouses of enzymes that revitalize and regenerate your entire body. These refreshing juices send forth cleansing catalysts that penetrate the innermost recesses of your body and dislodge the accumulated grit and pollutants from your cells and organs. At the same time, the juices are rich in nutrients that can repair your vital tissues and organs and help give you the look and feel of youth, no matter what your age.

CAUSE OF AGING: CELLULAR GRIME

To understand the importance of cleansing with raw juices, you need to know the basic cause of aging and how to reverse this health threat. Aging occurs when your biological process of cell regeneration becomes sluggish. What causes this slowdown? The accumulation of grime and sediment in your tissues. These pollutants block cellular nourishment. Denied essential elements, your cells start to wither and die. This is the root cause of your aging.

Cells Need Cleaning and Nourishment You are a magnificent package of cells. Each one is an independent unit with its individual metabolism. It needs to be kept clean and nourished. It must have a constant supply of life-giving oxygen. If there is any accumulation of rust-like plaque that clings to the membrane and cellular interior, a clogging of the free flow of both oxygen and nourishment will occur. This causes cellular disintegration. If too many of your cells are allowed to die in the polluted overload, the aging process proceeds at a steady rate. You can see it in the form of aging skin. You can feel it in the form of tiredness and recurring illness. To nip this in the bud, you need to use juices to invigorate your cells with cleansing and nourishment.

RAW JUICES ARE SWIFT IN CELLULAR REGENERATION

You need swift cellular cleansing. Your cells are in a constant dying-replacement rhythm. If more cells break down and die than are rebuilt, the aging process occurs all the quicker. *Caution:* The aged and decaying cells decompose rapidly. To prevent their accumulation and clogging, you need to eliminate them as quickly as possible from your system. *Remedy:* Fresh juices will help rebuild these cells and also wash out the decayed and dead ones so they do not become accumulated refuse in your body.

Cleanses, Rebuilds, Revitalizes   Within moments after you consume a glass of your favorite raw juice, the nutrients and enzymes go to work to create this internal rejuvenation. The juice nutrients speed up the biological process of cleansing away the dead and decaying cells. Immediately, the same juice nutrients stimulate and hasten the building of new cells. When the toxic waste products that have been blocking cellular oxygenation and nourishment are washed out, then the juices accelerate the normal metabolic and cell-rebuilding rates. These remarkable results take place in a short time, thanks to the super-power of raw juice elements.

JUICES WORK FASTER THAN WHOLE FOODS

When the liquid portion is extracted from the fruit or vegetable, it becomes a highly concentrated source of super cleansing without comparison. The juice is rapidly assimilated by your digestive system, requiring virtually no digestive action. For this reason, you will feel an instant "lift" when drinking a glass of orange juice, swifter than if you eat the whole fruit.

Whole fruits and vegetables that are thoroughly chewed are

extremely valuable sources of nutrients and cleansing elements. They should be enjoyed daily for inner and outer regeneration. But for swift action on cellular scrubbing, raw juices should also be enjoyed. Together, the combination can help you enjoy a prolonged "prime of life" at any age.

SEVEN CLEANSING-REJUVENATING POWERS OF FRESH JUICES

Fresh raw fruit or vegetable juices offer these immediate rewards in cleansing and rejuvenating.

1. *Nutritional Regeneration.* Free of the pulp, the rich juices are high concentrations of vitamins, minerals, trace elements, enzymes, and other elements that work speedily to create nutritional regeneration and cleansing of your entire body.

2. *Quick Assimilation.* In liquid form, these valuable cleansing elements are assimilated quickly into your bloodstream. As juices, they do *not* require digestive effort, hence their "instant" assimilation and cleansing activity. These juices do not interfere with other digestive activities, and pose no "load" on your system.

3. *Bypass Hydrochloric Acid.* Fresh juices do not call for the use of hydrochloric acid, which often causes cellular disintegration, if used in excess. Spare your digestive system the outpouring of this harsh and volatile acid; juices can perform without distress or discomfort.

4. *Total Package of Cleansing.* The concentrated nutritive elements create a stabilizing of your basic biological processes so that cleansing and regeneration are more effectively consummated. Juice nutrients are so perfectly balanced by nature that they speed up the regenerative process almost at the start.

5. *Balances Acid-Alkaline Levels.* Vegetable juices are dynamic sources of alkaline reserve. This helps give you an important acid-alkaline balance in your bloodstream and your tissues. This eases distress and also helps wash away the corrosive destruction of your vital organs.

6. *Improves Mineral Nourishment.* Adequate concentrations of minerals in the fruits and vegetables will help restore the biochemical and mineral balance in your bloodstream, organs, cells, tissues.

Special Benefit: A mineral deficiency is usually the forerunner of oxygen loss which then "chokes" and "starves" your cells and causes waste buildup. With juices, minerals provide oxygen and nourishment and accelerate the cleansing process.

7. *Speeds Up Cleansing Method.* Fresh raw juices contain powerful enzymes which alert the *micro-electric tension factor* in your body. This speeds up the cleansing of your cells and organs. At the same time, this factor creates a "magnet" action whereby nutrients are absorbed from your bloodstream to nourish your internal organs. This same "magnet" action effectively discharges metabolic refuse.

The best indication of the cleansing-healing power of juices is when you finish one or two glasses of a freshly prepared beverage. You feel so refreshed, alert, and good all over. That is the "instant" cleansing power of fresh juices.

Selecting Your Fruits, Vegetables   Fruits and vegetables should be fresh, seasonal, and free of decay. If you notice any signs of deterioration, then just cut away that portion and discard.

Wash all fruits and vegetables before you juice them. Use free-flowing cold water from your kitchen faucet. If you prefer, use a scrub brush for your vegetables to make certain that all dirt or debris has been removed.

If possible, juice your fruits or vegetables the same day you bring them home from the market. Otherwise, store in the crisper of your refrigerator. Do *not* cut until ready to juice, since this causes loss of important cleansing elements and nutrients.

Easy Way to Prepare Juice   You may use a hand juicer or an electric product. These are available at health stores and housewares outlets. Just cut up the fruit or vegetable and insert in your juicer.

Plan to use the juice right away. You may store overnight in a closed container in your refrigerator even though a small amount of the nutrients will evaporate. Use squeezed juice within two days, though, to derive maximum benefits.

Do Not Combine Fruit with Vegetable Juice   Fruit enzymes and nutrients are of a different density than those found in vegetables. If combined, there is a diluting of these elements and the cleansing-regenerative abilities are subsequently weakened. Therefore, combining them is a "no-no."

Feel free to combine any seasonal fresh fruits, if desired, for a tasty juice that will work without upset. Also, it is fine to combine different seasonal vegetables to make a beverage that is powerful in cleansing.

SIMPLE JUICE-TAKING PROGRAM

Plan to consume about three to four glasses of juices daily on this easy program. *Before Breakfast:* A glass of fresh fruit juice. *Noontime:* A glass of fresh vegetable juice after your meal. *Mid-Afternoon:* A glass of fresh fruit juice. *Dinnertime:* A glass of fresh fruit *or* vegetable juice after your meal. *Nightcap:* A glass of fresh vegetable juice. This helps you sleep better, too, through mineralization of your system.

This simple program will nourish your body and provide around-the-clock cleansing-regenerating nutrients to make you look and feel in great shape.

Gets Rid of 30 Years for 30¢ in Three Days

Crepe-like skin, hangdog look, poor memory, shaking hands, and chronic fatigue made Ida DiN. fearful of having to look in the mirror. When someone erringly thought she was her daughter's grandmother, she was spurred into action. She asked a health spa dietician about a program to offer help for aging. The dietician said countless people were able to roll back the clock on a raw juice fast. For just three days, she was to consume no food, but just drink juices. The first day, all fruit juices. The second day, all vegetable juices. The third day, all fruit juices. Ida DiN. dragged herself to a nearby wholesaler and bought a supply of fresh produce. She tried the program. Instantly, her skin firmed up, she sparkled with vitality, had improved memory, firm hands, and boundless energy. In just three days, she looked as if she had shed 30 years, and all for just 30¢ per day, which was the cost of the juices! She had used juices to scour her body and make herself brand new, within and without.

TASTY JUICES FOR HEALING OF COMMON AILMENTS

Everyday fruits and vegetables offer cleansing elements that create quick healing of common ailments. The juices are tasty and the results are dynamically effective.

Carrot Juice for Digestive System Cleansing   The rich concentration of Vitamin A and fiber residue in carrot juice combine to work swiftly to speed up digestive-intestinal cleansing. These combined nutrients do more than liquefy and dilute wastes; they speed up their removal. These nutrients further boost bile acid removal and also cleanse the colon. The entire region of your digestive-eliminative system will be cleansed and super-charged with vitality when you enjoy one or two glasses of carrot juice daily.

Intestine Cleanser   Try several glasses daily of cabbage juice. It contains factors that wash away the plaque clinging to your intestines. These factors also dilute the hydrochloric acid and protect against ulcer formation and burning. Cabbage juice will also cleanse wounds in the stomach lining and promote healing to help you overcome ulcerous infections.

Cooling Off Internal Inflammation   Tangy cranberry juice cleanses your bloodstream and then helps to acidify your urine which will protect against *dysuria* (painful elimination) and disorders of the prostate gland and the bladder. Painful voiding is eased when cranberry juice washes away irritating wastes and induces a soothing and natural release.

Juice Corrects Kidney Inflammation

In a reported situation, a 66-year old woman, Mabel O'H. was troubled with kidney inflammation for five years. Diagnosed as chronic pyelonephritis, she submitted to drugs, antibiotics, painful dilations, but with no help. She was put on a cranberry juice program, and was to drink two six-ounce glassfuls daily. After eight weeks, her urine gradually began to clear. At the end of nine months, there were only occasional pus cells. She continued on with the simple cranberry juice program because it helped her overcome kidney inflammation when drugs did not.

Apple Juice as Virus-Cleanser   Fresh apple juice contains a virus-fighting substance that is able to cleanse away dangerous germs. These substances combine with the virus during transit through the digestive system, help to "knock it out," and speed the elimination of the virus. Several glasses throughout the week will help wash away virus infestations and protect you against molecular deterioration caused by these wastes.

Dissolve Mucus with Pineapple Juice   Freshly prepared pineapple juice contains a digestive enzyme called bromelain. This is a powerful mucus washer. It actually works to dissolve the mucus waste and prepare it for elimination. Mucus is not only in your respiratory-bronchial tract but in various parts of your body. It is waste that clings together. It can be discharged and eliminated with powerful pineapple juice.

Washes Away Gastric Wastes in Three Months

At age 57, Rose A.Q. started to throw up and complain of post-dinner distress. Tests showed she had a thick accumulation of wastes in her stomach. (Called a *bezoar*, or ball-like mass, it lodged in her digestive system.) Her physician had administered meat tenderizer to dissolve the waste mass but it caused so much burning that it had to be stopped. Then she was told to take about 10 ounces of plain pineapple juice, three times a day, 30 minutes before each meal. In eight weeks, x-rays showed the bezoar had shrunk to half its original size. A few weeks later, the threatening waste mass was gone! This mucus glue had been dissolved through the action of the bromelain in the pineapple juice. She was healed and all this happened in less than three months.

Vegetable Juices Cleanse Bacteria   There are eight vegetables whose juices contain a powerful waste cleansing enzyme called *lysozyme*. When you drink juices made from these vegetables (singly or in combination) you send forth the lysozyme cleanser, which ingests bacteria and foreign particles and prepares them for expulsion. You are rewarded with a cleaner and healthier body, free of harmful bacteria. These eight vegetable juices are made from: cauliflower, cabbage, red radish, white radish, turnip, parsnip, broccoli, rutabaga. *Suggestion:* You may blenderize these vegetables into a puree and have a powerful bacteria-cleansing raw juice. The slight pulp in the puree adds sweeping fiber that doubles the cleansing action.

You *can* drink your way to a cleaner body and a healthier way of living. You can roll back the years as you wash out your wastes with raw juices, your rivers of super health.

IN REVIEW

1. Fresh raw juices cleanse your cells and organs as they promote regeneration and rebuilding of your various systems.

2. Note the seven cleansing-rejuvenating powers of fresh juices.
3. Ida DiN. washed away 30 years of aging for just 30¢ in juices in three days.
4. Mabel O'H. corrected kidney inflammation on a cranberry juice program.
5. Rose A.Q. dissolved waste lumps in her stomach and avoided surgery with the use of simple pineapple juice. All natural, all within three months.

CHAPTER 18

A Treasury of Cleansing Programs for Common and Uncommon Everyday Problems

Everyday foods, simple exercises, inhalation, and tasty homemade tonics all have the ability to dislodge the accumulated wastes in your system and prepare them for elimination. Once your vital organs and systems have been cleansed, you are able to enjoy a speedy healing for many internal and external health problems.

Here is a mini-listing of everyday health problems that can be traced to toxic accumulation. The simple cleansers work almost at once. They help correct the common (or uncommon) problem so that you can enjoy effective healing and a feeling of clean rejuvenation.

High Blood Pressure   The use of everyday garlic, either a clove or two as part of a salad or in cooking, can help control your pressure. Garlic has a dilating effect on your blood vessels and cleanses away the blockages that prevent free blood flow and contribute to arterial narrowing and a rise in blood pressure. Use garlic daily to promote cleansing and balancing of pressure.

Acne   Boost your intake of foods and juices high in the cleansing Vitamins A and D. These include fish liver oils, carrots, broccoli, sun-dried apricots, cantaloupe, desiccated liver, Vitamin D-fortified milk. These vitamins help cleanse the sebaceous glands of waste-filled oils that clog and plug pores, giving rise to blemishes.

Arthritis   This disabling ailment is often traced to an imbalance of calcium and phosphorus. This disturbance can be caused by sediment that blocks the free metabolic process of these nutrients. Cleanse debris by taking bone meal (available in tablet or powder form from health stores) daily as part of a total cleansing program.

Atherosclerosis   Also known as hardening of the arteries, this problem is caused by excessive cholesterol and fatty waste accumulations. To cleanse, boost your intake of lecithin, a fat-melting soybean product (available in health stores) and limit intake of animal foods.

Three Day Artery Cleansing

Advised by her nutritionist to follow a three-day artery cleansing regimen, Bernice L. simply *omitted* all animal-source foods. She took four tablespoons of lecithin daily, in her vegetable juices, sprinkled over salads, baked in meatless loaves, even added to soups. Bernice L. was then found to have "clean arteries."

Rheumatic Inflammation   Similar to arthritis, the excessive throbbing heat that is often felt is the result of chafing, irritating debris that clings to the skeletal and venous structure. To cleanse, include garlic in your daily food plan. *Simple:* Chew two or three cloves daily, and mask the odor with parsley, cloves, or cinnamon. Garlic is an excellent detoxifier and it boosts the general metabolism and stimulates your cleansing reaction. It helps ease and erase the toxic cause of rheumatic inflammation, often in days.

Sores, Wounds   Swift healing is possible when you mix freshly grated garlic with olive oil as a poultice. Apply directly to the sores or blemishes for several days. Massage very gently. The toxic-fighting ingredients in the garlic and the essential fatty acids of the olive oil help cleanse away infectious bacteria and restore cellular integrity and swift clearing.

Breathing Difficulties   Whether an allergy, sensitivity, or congestion, the aim is to cast out the accumulated wastes that cling to the delicate fibers of your respiratory organs. A simple remedy is to stand before an open window (be careful of drafts, though) and breathe in through your nostrils very deeply. Think of your lungs as balloons. Fill up to the brim! Hold it for the count of 10. Then exhale slowly through your mouth. Repeat five times. This deep breathing helps sweep away toxic wastes that are choking your lungs and causing many breathing difficulties.

Mouth Sores   Fragile oral tissues split and remain broken because the membranes have become clogged with wastes. You need to rebuild your mouth tissues. The use of bioflavonoids (found in citrus fruits and their juices; use the white membranous strings which are highly concentrated in these cleansing-rebuilding nutrients) will help heal this condition speedily.

Fever Blisters   With these pus-filled blisters, the object here is to cleanse away these toxic waste clumps. *Simple Remedy:* Dip a cotton swab into a bit of ether (from pharmacist) and apply to the blister. It "destroys" the toxic germs and helps remove them. Within moments, the blister or cold sore will start to heal.

Constipation   Weakened or inactive bowels become choked with stubborn waste deposits. To cleanse them, activate your sphincter muscles through the use of the all-natural prune or fig juice (or a combo). Just one or two glasses in the morning helps "knock out" the bacterial blockages and boost their removal, almost at once.

Cramps   Whether in your legs, arms, back, or anywhere else, cramps can be debilitating. They indicate that bacteria wastes are "locked in" your skeletal and musculature structures. A danger here is that they "devour" calcium and this leads to the cramps. To win this battle, just drink one or two glasses of milk. (Skim, if you are fat-calorie watching.) The rich concentration of calcium will help strengthen these pockets and thereby "chase" out wastes. In many situations, it works overnight!

Ends Lifelong Cramps Battle with One Home Remedy

Severe body cramps, especially upon awakening, made Allen T. feel like an invalid. It took him an hour to "untie the knots" through careful walking. But the pains always returned in a few days! A metabolic physician (specialist in whole body treatments) said that infectious wastes had lodged in muscular pockets and were causing the congestion. A simple suggestion: boost intake of cleansing and restoring calcium through just one or two glasses of milk, especially at night time. Allen T. tried it. Miraculously, the next morning the pains were gone. Thanks to the cleansing calcium, he never again had the cramps that had otherwise been plaguing him for a lifetime.

Stress, Tension   You know the symptoms: you cannot relax; you're high-strung. The reason for this is that debris tends to grate and chafe at your nerves. Cleanse away this irritating toxemia, and you will feel soothed all over. Do this with a simple "rag doll" approach. Lie down in a bed. Let yourself go. Concentrate on releasing all tightness from the tips of your fingers to the top of your head. Make yourself as limp as a dishrag. *Tip:* Your head should be able to roll easily from side to side. If you have any stiffness or resistance, you have not quite mastered relaxation. Keep on making yourself limp through the power of your thoughts. In so doing, the tight pockets of wastes will be dislodged and evaporated in a short time. Just 30 minutes daily of this "rag doll" approach will wash away stress-causing wastes and make you feel contented and happy.

Headaches   Wash away irritating debris caused by caffeine and tannic acids by eliminating such beverages (coffee, cola, commercial teas) and switching to fresh fruit and vegetable juices. They contain healthy nutrients and cleansing enzymes that will uproot and sweep away the nerve-irritating caffeine wastes.

Stomach Upset   Use a clove of garlic, chewed raw or diced for a salad. Just a little bit is enough to create a magical soothing. Garlic is a prime source of a waste-cleanser known as gasteoenteric allichalon which is able to wash away debris from the motor activation center of your stomach. Within moments, the cleansing restores comfort and eases upset. It's a natural stomach tonic.

For Women Only   The monthly pain women are resigned to endure can often be traced to toxic wastes that need to be removed. The hormonal influences that prompt a monthly cycle can be damaged if bacterial sludge acts as a barrier to the natural process. To cleanse away these barricades, two remedies are effective. (1) In a glass of fresh fruit juice, add 1 tablespoon of brewer's yeast powder (from any health store). Stir vigorously or blenderize. Drink slowly. It is a powerhouse of enzymes and Vitamin C and B-complex vitamins. These converge upon wastes and uproot and eliminate them. There is a soothing contentment felt almost at once. (2) With the approach of the monthly period, wastes pool together and tend to displace valuable blood calcium. This mineral is a powerful cleanser and pain reliever. Just use calcium supplements or skim milk in moderate amounts. Blood calcium levels are balanced quickly and wastes are washed out and contentment restored.

Rectal Itching This embarrassing problem can be blamed upon venous congestion, especially with wastes from white sugar and white flour products. Chemical residues accumulate in the veins and arteries of the groin and cause the nagging itch. To correct, simply eliminate all foods containing sugar and bleached flour. You'll become cleaner and itch-free almost at once.

Acid (Sour) Stomach This is also known as heartburn. Its cause is often traced to excessive accumulation of acid-producing byproducts. Reduce wastes by avoiding alcohol, coffee, tea, tobacco, and most animal-source foods. The potato creates an alkaline reaction in the body that helps neutralize stomach acidity and knock out the irritating acidic wastes. Plan to boost intake of potatoes (without salt or fatty dressing) and feel your stomach cleansing itself and becoming "sweet" again.

Colds, Winter Ailments Bacterial infections need to be cleansed away. For centuries, garlic has been used to ease problems such as sore throat, runny nose, fever, cough. Just chew on one or two garlic cloves during the day and you'll help detoxify your system and conquer your colds quickly.

HOW JUICES GIVE YOU QUICK CLEANSING AND BETTER HEALTH

Fresh fruit and vegetable juices are assimilated rapidly so that their nutrients and enzymes can cleanse your cells and pave the way for improved health. Here is a listing of the most common juices for healing common and uncommon health disorders.

Apple Juice. Improves elimination; helps cleanse skeletal structure; loosens blockages to help correct digestive disorders.

Apricot Juice. A prime source of highly concentrated vitamins, minerals, and enzymes, needed to purify the bloodstream and regenerate the circulatory system.

Beet Juice. Very potent so combine it with other vegetables such as celery, cucumber, lettuce, cabbage. Its action purifies your bloodstream and cleanses your nervous system.

Blackberry Juice. Combine with equal amounts of fresh water and drink it in the morning to initiate peristalsis, which then promotes regularity. It's a healthy cleanser.

Blueberry Juice. Its prime concentration of bioflavonoids helps stabilize your digestive system; it also soothes problems such as colitis, diarrhea, intestinal infections. *Tip:* When troubled with excessive amounts of uric acid, a waste product, drink blueberry juice. It acts as a natural cleanser of this waste.

Carrot Juice. Helps cleanse vital organs and neutralize circulating blood impurities, not to mention waste-causing skin blemishes. It is a prime source of carotene (a predecessor to Vitamin A), which is needed to improve the health of your skin through cleansing actions.

Celery Juice. Take it alone or mixed with other vegetable juices (and a squeeze of lemon). It helps cleanse the liver and kidneys, and also washes impurities out of the bloodstream. It is also said to help wash the nervous system and cleanse the adrenal glands.

Cherry Juice. The unusually rich concentration of both bioflavonoids and enzymes make this a high-energy drink. It helps wash away the cells and tissues, protecting against waste-causing aging. It appears to protect against arthritis.

Cucumber Juice. A refreshing drink, its mildness should not be deceiving. It acts as a powerful solvent of uric acid, the waste that can cause illnesses. Take it pure or combine with carrot and/or celery juice. It washes away debris in a matter of hours.

Currant Juice. Whether made from black or red currants, this juice is a powerful source of organ cleansers. Waste products that might clog liver and digestive organs are washed away with the enzymes and nutrients in this tasty juice.

Grape Juice. Rich in natural fruit sugars, it helps raise your energy levels in minutes. It is also able to cleanse away impurities, preventing formation of stones. It boosts the excretion of urea, thereby relieving internal congestion. If you use bottled or canned grape juice, make certain it is free of added sugar.

Grapefruit Juice. Its powerful nutrients stimulate the flow of bile, thereby improving the health of your liver. It cleanses your tissues and cells so that wastes cannot destroy capillaries.

Lemon Juice. This is very potent, so you would not want to take more than two or three tablespoons as part of a citrus juice combo. Its Vitamin C and minerals tend to cleanse blood impurities and protect against infectious allergies and respiratory distress.

Lettuce Juice. The rich concentration of cleansing nutrients helps wash away wastes from organs to prevent spasms and grating irritation.

Orange Juice. A tasty juice, its vitamins help cleanse your blood plasma of impurities and strengthen your vascular walls. Especially cleansing are the bioflavonoids found in the pulp. Use it all.

Peach Juice. Promotes natural urination to wash away stored up wastes.

Pear Juice. Its ingredients are able to scrub bowels and kidneys and its minerals also help regenerate your blood cells.

Pineapple Juice. A near-miracle juice rich in scrubbing enzymes that are able to uproot the most stubborn of wastes. It is a powerful cleanser for vital organs.

Tomato Juice. It should be salt-free to provide important minerals and enzymes that help cleanse the bloodstream, correct arterial health, and guard against cellular deterioration.

Suggestion   Take fresh juices daily to help keep your system as clean as possible. You will be rewarded with protection against ailments and a lifestyle that will be filled with energy and vitality.

You can be healthier, look younger, live longer, and have a sparklingly clean body, inside and outside. With the use of these everyday foods, you can rebuild your life and enjoy a sludge-free, longer life span. Free yourself from joint-muscle-artery-circulation sludge and discover a world of "eternal youth," beginning right now!

SUMMARY

1. Clear up any ailments with the use of everyday foods and simple healers that promote internal-external cleansing in minutes.

2. Bernice L. overcame the risk of atherosclerosis on a simple three-day artery-cleansing system.

3. Allen T. freed himself from his lifelong cramps battle with one home remedy that worked overnight.

4. Fresh juices act as powerhouses in detoxifying your system and promoting youthful well-being. They are refreshingly good, too.

Index

A

Acetylcholine 104–105
Aches 143–150
Acid (Sour) stomach 183
Acne 179–180
ADP 100, 103–104, 106
Aging 171–178
"Aging Stiffness" 103–109
"All-Natural Heart Cleansing Tonic" 92–93
Allergies 77–84
Allicin 31, 139
Allisotin 24
Apple 34
Arteries 53–54, 133–141
Arteriosclerosis 29–30, 134, 135
Atherosclerosis 180
ATP 74–75
Arthritis 19–28, 180

B

Bacteria, cleansing of 177
Balloon Breathing 129–130
Bile 30
Bioflavonoids 114–116
Blood pressure 51–59
Bloodstream 125–131
Body Motions 140, 143–150
Bran 164–168
Breathing 44
Breathing difficulties 180–181
Breathing, problems of 77–84
Bronchial tubes 78–79
Bulk 161–169
Bursitis 144–146

C

"C+Iron Tonic" 129
Cabbage juice 66
Caffeine 57
Carbohydrates, refined 138
Cell-slimming 70–71
Cell-washing 127–129
Cells, body 151–159
Cells, overload of 69–70, 74–76
Cells, washing of 77–84
Cellular grime 171–172
Cellular regeneration 172
Cellulite 41–46
Chewing 67
Cholesterol, 29–40, 135
Cholesterol, chart of 37–39
Cholesterol, overload of 36–37
Choline 31–32
Circulation 95–102
Circulation, foods that block 98–99
Citrus juices, 153–155
Clots, waste-filled 99–100
Colds 183
Collagen 153
Constipation, 61, 63, 181
Cramps 181
Cranberry juice 120

D

Detoxification 95–96
Diallyldisulfide 31
Digestive system 61–68
Digestive system, cleansing of 176

E

EPA 22–34
"Early Morning Circulation Booster" 97–98
Ears 116–118
Eating, methods of 65
Enzymatic catalysts 87–88, 96
Enzymes 43, 70–71, 171
Exercise, 26–28, 35, 45, 57, 106–107, 137–138, 143–150
Eyes 111–116

F

Fast, one-day grape juice 96–97
Fast, one-day juice 78–79
Fast, raw food 73–74
Fat 134
Fats 56
Fats, animal 65, 138–139, 155–156
Feet, aches in 149–150
Fever blisters 181
Fiber 161–169
Fiber, food sources of 164–165
Food, raw 73
Foods, high enzyme 71–73
Foods, waste-causing 75–76
Foods, waste-cleansing 86–87
Foods, waste-forming 86–87
Fruits 20, 34

G

Gallbladder 121–124
Gallbladder crystals 122–123
Gallstones 121–122
Garlic 23–25, 30–31, 53–55, 57–58, 63–64, . 88–89, 107–108, 126–127, 139
Gastrointestinal tract, 162–163

H

HDL-LDL 32–35
Headaches 182
Hearing 116–118
Hearing, diet for super- 117–118

Heart, 85–94, 135
High blood pressure 179
Hydrotherapy 25–26
Hypertension 51–59

I

Indigestion 64–66
Inflammation, internal 176
"Instant Power Potion" 105–106
Interferon 158
Intestine, cleanser 176
Iron 127–129

J

Joints 103–109
Joints, steam cleaning of 108
Juice, raw 171–178

K

Kidneys 118–120
Kidneys, gravel in 120
Kidneys, washing of debris in 119–120

L

LCAT 90
Lactic acid 104
Lecithin 31–32, 89–91, 104–106
Legs, cramps in 146–147
Liver 29
Liver, washing of 120–121
Lymph system 156–159

M

"Magic Drink" 66–67
Massage 44
Metabolism, sluggish 139–141
Minerals 112, 136
Monthly tensions 182–183
"Miracle Salad" 63–64

Mouth sores 181
"Morning Bran Booster Tonic" 166–167
Mucus 176–177

N

Nearsightedness 112–113
Nightshade foods 21–22
Nostrils, alternate breathing of 82–83

O

Octacosanol 140, 167
Oil, cod liver 22–23
Oils, fish 156–159
Onions 54–55, 91–92
Organs, vital 111–124
Overweight 69–76
Oxygen 137–138

P

Pain 143–150
Pectin 32–34
Pollutants 79-80
Pollution, indoor 80–81
Potassium 56, 62
Prune 62–63

R

Raw food plan 20–21
Rectal itching 183
Regularity 43–44
Rejuvenating 173–174
Rheumatoid inflammation 180
Roughage 43–44, 64
Roughage, food sources 161–169

S

Salt 55–56
"Sight-Saving Tonic" 115–116
Skin, 41–50, 46–49

Skin, blemishes 46–49
Smoking 3ᴦ
Sores 180
"Steam Cleaning" 25–26
Stomach, upset 182
Stress 182
Stretching 26–28
Sugar 111–113
Supplements 136

T

Tension 45, 182
Thermostat, internal 25–26
Thromboxane 54–55
Toxemia 85–94, 112–113
Toxic wastes 19–20, 52–53
Triglyceride 128–139
"Triple-Action Blood-Washing Potion"
      130–131
"Triple Circulation Pick-Up Elixir" 101–102

U

Ulcers 66–68

V

Vegetables 20
Virus cleanser 176
Vitamin B6 100–101
Vitamin C 114–116, 152–155
Vitamin D 158–159

W

Wastes, fatty 69–76
Weight 57
Wheat germ 167–168
Wheat germ oil 140
Whistling 83
Whitaker, M.D., Julian 135–137
Winter ailments 183
"Wonder Youth Tonic" 154–155
Wounds 180